SEX OVER 40

ALSO BY SAUL H. ROSENTHAL, M.D.

Sex Over 40

SEX OVER 40

COMPLETELY REVISED AND UPDATED

SAUL H. ROSENTHAL, M.D.

Jeremy P. Tarcher / Putnam

A member of Penguin Putnam Inc. / New York

Most Tarcher/Putnam books are available at special quantity discounts for bulk purchases for sales promotions, premiums, fund-raising, and educational needs. Special books or book excerpts also can be created to fit specific needs. For details, write Putnam Special Markets, 375 Hudson Street, New York, NY 10014.

Jeremy P. Tarcher/Putnam
a member of
Penguin Putnam Inc.
375 Hudson Street
New York, NY 10014
www.penguinputnam.com

Originally published as *The New Sex Over 40*

First trade paperback edition 2000

Copyright © 1999 by Saul H. Rosenthal, M.D.

Library of Congress Cataloging-in-Publication Data

Rosenthal, Saul H.
Sex over 40 / Saul H. Rosenthal.
p.   cm.
ISBN 1-58542-054-9
1. Sex instruction.   2. Middle aged persons—Sexual behavior.   I. Title.
HQ31.R8433   2000   00-056772

Printed in the United States of America

9   10

Book design by Chris Welch

This book is dedicated to my wife,
Cindy, who has been
my inspiration, playmate, and best friend,
and to my little daughter,
Sadie, who has been a source of
never-ending delight to me.

CONTENTS

ACKNOWLEDGMENTS

Just as I did in the first edition of this book, I have to start off by acknowledging the debt I owe to the many patients who have provided the foundation of my knowledge about sexual function and dysfunction. Without my experience in helping them, this book could not have been written.

Next, I have to thank my wife, Cindy, who initially suggested I write a book about sex over forty and who has been my inspiration throughout. She also read the early versions of most of the chapters and made many useful suggestions.

I have been amazed by the cooperation and helpfulness of my colleagues in other fields of medicine who patiently took time out of their busy practices to be of assistance, answer my questions, and read over draft versions of chapters for correctness of information as it applied to their fields. I would especially like to thank

Drs. William Fitch and Michael Newell in urology, Drs. José Trabal and Ely Nathan in gynecology, Dr. Gerald Rosenberg in rheumatology, Dr. Peter Ravdin in oncology, and Drs. Charles Roeth and Chris Kopecky in cardiology. I also consulted, although more briefly, with Drs. Irwin Goldstein and Jennifer Berman with regard to the effects of Viagra on women.

I also really appreciate my editor at Tarcher, Mitch Horowitz, who was very supportive of the idea of an updated edition of this book from the first and who has been helpful and easy to work with throughout!

In the first edition, I had to thank my secretary who typed draft after draft with needed corrections. For this edition it only seems right to conclude my acknowledgments by thanking my word processor, which made the whole process so easy.

WHY A BOOK ABOUT
SEX OVER FORTY?

So often in my practice, men and women over forty—good, solid, respectable men and women like yourselves—came to me at the point of desperation. They were afraid that their sexual lives were declining to extinction, and they didn't really understand what was happening or what could be done. When they were in sexual situations these men and women felt humiliated, embarrassed, rejected, helpless, or just plain disappointed. It's easy to feel like a failure or to feel that you've lost your masculinity or femininity when sex isn't working.

It's tragic that this happens so frequently. These years should bring the most satisfying sexual experiences of a person's life and bolster feelings of self-esteem and successfulness. In fact, many of the older men and women I treated found that when their sexual lives were restored *the rest of their lives* became meaningful again.

There has supposedly been a "sexual revolution," and there is certainly a lot more sexual information available now than there was twenty or thirty years ago. Until very recently, however, almost all this information continued to be addressed to young adults. It has always been difficult for men and women like us, who are over forty, fifty, or sixty, to find sexual information intended specifically *for us*—information that could help us understand the changes in *our* sexual lives.

At this point in our lives we have different sexual needs and sexual problems from people in their twenties and thirties. In spite of this, however, it has been very hard to find specialized sexual information that deals directly with our sexual wants, our needs, and our problems.

It has only been very recently, since the release of the remarkable new medication Viagra stimulated interest in the sexual problems that people our age face, that there has been more discussion of these issues. Yet even now, although one finds occasional articles and programs dealing with the sexual problems of older men and women, it's still difficult to find any comprehensive source of this information in one place.

I began teaching and practicing the treatment of sexual problems almost thirty years ago when I was a professor at the University of Texas Medical School here in San Antonio. My discussions with men and women like you showed me that there is a real need for a book about sex addressed directly to men and women our age. When I published the book *Sex Over 40* in 1987, many people called or wrote to thank me and tell me that that little book changed their lives. Now, however, it has become clear that with the new developments in the treatment of sexual dysfunction, and especially with the introduction of Viagra, there is a need for a new edition to incorporate these new developments—a *New Sex Over 40!*

The New Sex Over 40 is a reliable and up-to-date source of practical information that will help you to understand and adjust to your changing sexual responses. It can show you how to have a richer and more satisfying sexual life than you've ever had before, while teaching you how to adapt to the natural changes that are occurring in your body.

Many of us, especially those of us over fifty, were raised, and went through our sexually formative years, at a time when sexual information wasn't readily available at all. Undoubtedly our parents tried to teach us the various nonsexual skills that we needed to be healthy and successful people, but they usually omitted totally any education about how to be good sexual partners. It's very possible that they didn't really know themselves.

In fact, it's more than likely that your parents sheltered you from whatever limited information may have been available at the time. Thus your upbringing may well have left you with many inhibitions about expressing your sexuality.

When you did learn about sex you couldn't imagine "older" men and women, the age of your parents and grandparents, ever engaging in it. Now that you're their age yourself, you probably realize how childish that impression was. You're probably aware that sex is an important part of your life, and you're certainly not ready to see it vanish. Few of us are willing to lose the closeness, warmth, and intimacy that a good sexual relationship can bring.

As you get older you can't rely on sex just happening the way it did when you were younger. Men and women over forty and fifty undergo physical changes that, although normal and natural, affect their bodies' sexual responsiveness.

When you're over forty you can, and should, continue to have good, even wonderful, sexual experiences—but having them requires knowledge, adaptation, understanding, innovation, and imagination. You have to be aware of what's going on in your body and your partner's body. You need to adapt to these changes with a willing and enthusiastic use of your imagination—and with a spirit of innovation. You may also need to use some of the new medications and other treatments now available to help you adapt. (We'll discuss those in detail later.)

At this age your body may no longer "do its own thing" without much help, the way it did when you were younger. You and your partner need to work together now, more than ever, to get the most out of your sexual lives. It's now much more important for you to make love regularly, to use variation freely, and to avoid letting sex become routine or dull. In this book I'll help you find ways to express your sexuality that are both imaginative and sensible.

In addition to experiencing the normal physical changes that I've mentioned, men and women over forty are, unfortunately, more susceptible to a number of illnesses such as arthritis, high blood pressure, heart conditions, and diabetes that can affect their sexuality. If you have one of these conditions, in addition to the sexual problems stemming from your illness you may also be required to take medications that have side effects that can add to your sexual difficulties.

Considering that the sexual changes of aging are universal and that the sexual consequences of illness are common for men and women over forty, it is absolutely astounding that relatively little has been written to guide older men and women with their specific sexual needs. I will attempt to fill this gap by supplying you with the most recent information on the sexual side effects of various illnesses and medications, as well as by suggesting the best ways to avoid these sexual problems.

In order to adapt to your changing body's responses and to sexual problems caused by illness you may need to vary the lovemaking activities that you usually use and the patterns of lovemaking to which you're accustomed.

Unfortunately, some older men and women were brainwashed with Victorian attitudes about sex during their early years. The resulting closed-mindedness causes them to feel that they have few options available—that any sexual variation from whatever they have been doing for the last twenty-five years is probably immoral, perverse, or a sign of inadequacy. Thus, their upbringing not only limits their knowledge of sexual options and variations; it has also left them with many inhibitions about what is right, proper, and appropriate.

Therefore, some older adults may be less flexible about adapting to changes in their bodies and overcoming sexual difficulties. In this book, I will suggest many ways for you to accommodate your lovemaking to the situations you may face—ways with which I hope almost anyone would feel comfortable.

WHY YOUR DOCTOR CAN'T ANSWER YOUR QUESTIONS ABOUT SEX

Your own physician may not have answers to your questions about how your body is functioning sexually. When I attended medical school at Harvard in the late fifties and early sixties, we were never taught anything about sex—nothing about sexual function or the treatment of sexual problems. In fact, at that time there weren't any courses about sex at medical schools anywhere in the country. Yet, when we physicians graduated from medical school, our patients came to us with sexual problems and expected us to be experts in the field.

Even now, although there has been a revolution in the scientific evaluation and treatment of sexual problems, these subjects have managed to win a very small place, if any, in most medical schools' curricula. Doctors may be taught how to do the surgery to install a penile implant, for instance, but that is not the same as learning about sexual function. It's therefore not surprising that so many doctors are uncomfortable talking about sexual problems. The truth is that they may know little more about the subject than their patients.

When you realize that most physicians were taught very little about sexual problems in medical school, their lack of interest in these problems becomes less surprising. They're busy working in their own fields, and they don't really have the time to acquire the specialized knowledge that's available on the treatment of sexual difficulties. For this reason, you are likely to find a wide range of knowledge and interest from one physician to another. Some doctors may be up on the latest research in diagnosis and treatment of sexual problems, while others may just not want to bother or may assign you to a treatment without much real thought.

I became interested in treating patients with sexual dysfunctions around 1970 because I realized what a tremendous need there was for sexual therapy. At that time, only a generation ago, treating sexual problems was considered a very daring thing to do. That in itself gives you an idea of how far we've come since then. In those years I was an associate professor of psychiatry at the University of Texas Medical School at San Antonio, but even as a professor one was risking his or her reputation by trying to treat and help people with sexual problems. At a time when even talking about sexual problems was considered risqué, actually treating these problems was felt by some to be almost indecent or salacious.

Nevertheless, at that time I also introduced the teaching of basic courses in sexuality, sexual function, and sexual treatment to the medical students at the university. Subsequently, I continued to treat men and women with sexual dysfunctions for more than twenty-five years, first at the university and then in private practice as the director of the Sexual Therapy Clinic of San Antonio. Although I am a psychiatrist, the program I used employed a comprehensive medical evaluation and treatment program that combined the skills of specialists in urology, endocrinology, gynecology, psychiatry, and other specialties.

Some years ago researchers didn't dare to apply science and technology to sexual problems for fear of being labeled charlatans. In the past twenty years, however, that situation has radically changed. From a scientific viewpoint, at least, the medical establishment's era of neglect of the topic of sexual dysfunction is over. The first advances were in the diagnosis of sexual problems. They began in the 1970s and combined medicine and technology in a wide array of diagnostic techniques ranging from hormonal and blood chemistry tests to the measurement of nighttime erections and the blood pressure of the penis.

These advances in diagnosis were accompanied by the development of new treatments. For instance, at the time I wrote the first edition of this book in the mid-1980s, the treatments that were available for impotence included penile implants, mechanical vacuum devices, penile injections, and a few medicines and herbs with only mild to moderate effectiveness.

In the past ten years, however, the pharmaceutical industry has awakened to this promising field. Pharmaceutical research now is going full tilt, and the first really effective medicine, Viagra, was introduced in 1999. This medicine and others in the pipeline will create a new "sexual revolution" for men and women over forty.

Twenty-five years ago, the latest advance in treating sexual dysfunction was nonmedical "sexual therapy" based on the Masters and Johnson approach. This was far better than anything that had come before, but now, sexual therapy, without medical evaluation and treatment, is simply no longer acceptable or adequate.

I've tried to write a book that presents the important sexual information you need in clear, straightforward, helpful, and inoffensive language. There is no section on HIV and other sexually transmitted diseases, as this subject is now touched on almost daily in the media. I felt that adequate coverage of it in this book would have taken space away from other material not so readily available to men and women over forty.

I hope that you will find many useful and helpful ideas in this book, and that it will help you to achieve a more open viewpoint about your sexuality. Different chapters will be meaningful to different people. Remember, however, that if you can find *one* important piece of information that will enrich your sexual life or help to restore your sexual functioning, it can revolutionize *your entire life.*

While this book is filled with practical information for you, the maximum benefit will come from sharing the book's ideas with your partner. Try to discuss the points that seem important to you. Doing so may help both of you to read the most pertinent sections of the book together.

In the past, the two of you may have felt awkward about discussing sex and may never have developed a vocabulary of sexual words you felt comfortable with. I hope that the book will help to provide both a vocabulary and a framework for talking about the sexual issues in your lives.

I also hope that you and your partner will enjoy this book, and that it will add to the richness and fullness of your life experiences.

PART

I

SEX AND THE
OVER-FORTY MALE

CHAPTER I

SEX AND THE OVER-FORTY MALE

Jack R. came into my office reluctantly. He looked embarrassed and depressed. A well-dressed, conservative-looking man in his early fifties, he was obviously accustomed to success in meeting life's challenges. Yet, he wasn't feeling successful about his sexual life, and he seemed extremely discouraged about it.

He had decided that he was "becoming impotent" and doubted if he could be helped. He said he often was unable to attain an erection. Moreover, the few times he did get hard, he would lose his erection before he climaxed.

Although Jack said that he was no longer getting erections, it soon became clear that he had a rather restricted definition of what that meant. What was actually happening was that he was no longer getting spontaneous erections—that is, he wasn't getting erect without stimulation of his penis. (And, as it turned out, his wife had been doing very little to provide the penile stimulation he needed in order to get erect.)

Jack's claim that he was losing his erections before climaxing was also misleading. Actually, he was maintaining his erections for quite a long time, but he was sometimes unable to climax, even with prolonged intercourse, and his erections would then gradually fade.

This man was unaware that what he was experiencing is quite common and to be expected for a man of his age. Unfortunately, he was still expecting his body to respond the same way it did twenty years ago, so his body's natural responses at fifty-plus had thrown him into a tailspin.

I've treated this same unwarranted anxiety in many over-forty men, and I've observed that it's usually lack of knowledge concerning sexual response after forty that produces such heightened anxiety and distress.

Some of the changes in your body that I'm going to tell you about may seem somewhat scary at first. You may not like to hear about them. But I'll also tell you how to deal with them successfully. Knowledge and a clear plan of how to respond to these changes are extremely important in maintaining an undiminished sex life as you get older.

When you're over forty, your penis may stop functioning the way you always expected it would. It may not get hard when you think it should, and it may act in other ways that are different from the ways you were used to in the past. If you start thinking that this means sex is almost over for you, or that your penis will soon stop functioning totally, it can be very frightening.

Many of our feelings of self-worth, self-esteem, and masculinity are tied to how we feel about ourselves sexually. If a man feels that he's failing sexually, that "he can't get it up," it's difficult for him to feel like a success in business, at home, or in any other area of his life. There's always that nagging feeling in the back of his mind that he's really not successful anymore.

If you're no longer getting erections whenever you want them, if they're not coming as spontaneously as you'd like, if sometimes you don't seem to have the need or ability to ejaculate, you may start having the same feelings Jack had—that your sexual ability is fading and that before long it will be gone. You've heard jokes and stories about sexually ineffective older men, and you may be frightened that you too are losing your sexual powers. This simply isn't true. Lovemaking doesn't have to diminish or end at forty, fifty, sixty—or any age. On the contrary, think of this as a time to *change your approach to sex*, rather than to give up on it, and you will learn to make your sexual life better than ever.

It's important to realize that the physical changes that occur throughout your body as you get older, while undeniable, don't require you to give up all the activities that you enjoy. Some physical things *you may even do better* than when you were in your twenties. If you've taken up jogging in recent years, for instance, you may run a lot more now—and be able to run much farther—than you could when you were younger.

It's the same with sex. By learning to adapt to change, you may find it possible to be an even better lover than before.

WHAT CAN YOU EXPECT?

Let's go over some of the natural bodily changes that occur as you get older. These changes are predictable and should neither surprise nor upset you.

You Will Need More Direct Stimulation in Order to Get Erect
One thing you can count on is that when you are over forty you
won't be getting spontaneous erections in the same rapid and easy
way you did when you were in your adolescence or early twenties.
At that age, just the thought of sex, seeing your undressed partner,
or a fantasy about a sexual situation would cause your penis to
spring to attention in a matter of seconds. This just isn't going to
happen anymore. As you mature, all the physiologic systems in
your body slow down—including this one.

You will, without a doubt, take longer and longer to become
erect from mental stimulation alone—just thinking about sex or
seeing a sexual partner won't be enough. You will require more and
more direct physical stimulation to your penis in order to get a
firm erection.

But that may not really be so bad. It certainly doesn't mean that
you're going to stop having erections or stop having sex. It just
means that your partner is going to have to help you get hard. And
here, an understanding, loving partner is truly important. She can
assist you by using her hands, her mouth, her breasts, or other
parts of her body to stimulate your penis—and this can open a
whole new chapter in your sex life, as your lovemaking becomes
more mutual, sensual, and varied.

Too often I've treated couples who didn't realize that an over-
forty man needs direct physical stimulation. In the past, his erections
had come spontaneously. The woman had rarely touched the man's
penis, and he had never really had a need for it. Now, gradually, he
was no longer getting spontaneous erections with any frequency. He
kept waiting for them, though, *before* approaching his wife. Their sexual encounters, therefore, became less and less frequent as he started
waiting a week, two weeks, then a month at a time, for that sponta-

neous erection that never came. Finally, the couple would come to see me, assuming that he was becoming impotent.

It's important to realize that you don't have to wait for an erection to start lovemaking. Your partner can help you get hard, and you can make love whenever the two of you desire.

You May Not Be Quite as Firm   A second change to be aware of is that your erections will lose some of the "rock-hard" firmness they had when you were younger. They will still, however, be more than adequate and firm enough so that you can enter your partner with ease and you can both enjoy full satisfaction.

Firmness is, for the most part, a cosmetic issue: While your penis may not be as hard as it used to be, it can still do the job very well. It's not how hard your penis is but how well you use it (and the rest of your body) that will determine how much you please your partner during lovemaking.

You'll Need to Climax Less Often   Many men over forty become concerned because they don't climax as readily or as easily as they used to, assuming this to be an early sign of impotence. One forty-eight-year-old patient of mine, Harold M., told me he was able to have intercourse, with a good erection, for almost thirty minutes at a time, but sometimes just wasn't able to get over the edge to climax. His complaint was that "the lovemaking really felt good, but it aggravated me that I couldn't come."

Instead of enjoying the experience, unfortunately, Harold allowed himself to get frustrated and annoyed. What he didn't realize was that as he had gotten older his body just didn't need to ejaculate as often as before. However, his frequency of intercourse hadn't significantly slowed—so now he was simply having intercourse more often than he needed to climax.

Masters and Johnson maintained that most men over sixty need only one or two climaxes per week. Some men cut down their frequency of lovemaking as they get older because of their decreased desire for ejaculation, but this isn't at all necessary. If you need a climax only once a week, you can still make love two or three times a week. You just have to be willing to adapt to the situation and to enjoy the many pleasures of lovemaking without pushing yourself to climax.

If you pressure yourself to climax when your body doesn't really need to, you may strain and strain and eventually lose your erection and then feel that the experience was a failure instead of a success. This can change what should be a very enjoyable experience into a tense and anxious one. You'll end up worrying about whether you'll be able to climax the next time you make love, and if you have trouble climaxing again you may even begin to fear attempting sex in the future.

Often my male patients feel that they're letting their partners down when they don't ejaculate. Sometimes a woman will feel that somehow she has failed sexually if her partner hasn't been able to reach a climax, that he no longer finds her attractive, or that he's been sleeping with somebody else.

Fifty-nine-year-old Henry B. came to my office desperate. He often was unable to climax during intercourse, and each time that happened it turned into a family catastrophe. His wife would cry and feel rejected and threatened. There was no way he could reassure her. He finally convinced her to come to the clinic with him for a consultation, and I explained to her that his occasional inability to ejaculate was due to his age rather than any lack of love for her.

Keep in mind that occasionally not climaxing is a natural occurrence after forty, one of the changes that you can easily adapt and adjust to. Lovemaking can be a very enjoyable sensual and sexual experience, with or without a climax. You don't need to climax every time you make love, and you shouldn't push yourself to. Just tell your partner in advance that you may not be able to climax so that she won't feel she's letting you down. Making love without that pressure to ejaculate can add a new dimension to your relationship, making it more pleasurable for you and your partner to enjoy leisurely and prolonged intercourse.

Another observation that I have made is that some men feel a sense of relief in not being so pushed and preoccupied with the *need* to climax so often. Phil, a fifty-five-year-old man, told me that "when I was younger, my body was always pressuring me for sex. I often couldn't think of anything else. Now I can pick and choose when I want to make love, at a time when I choose, instead of being constantly in need."

Lasting Longer, Enjoying More   Now that your body is no longer pressuring you for quick ejaculations, you'll probably be able to enjoy intercourse longer than you could when you were younger. This can be a real plus for your partner. Women often require longer stimulation in order to become fully aroused and to climax. Your partner will thus enjoy your newfound sexual endurance, and you'll both enjoy being able to continue with longer, more sensual lovemaking.

Waiting Time Between Erections   After climaxing, there is always a certain time period during which you are unable to get erect again. During this refractory period your penis will be unable to respond, no matter what the stimulation.

When you were in your early twenties, you probably could get a second erection just a few minutes after climaxing. That few-minute rest period probably lengthened to twenty minutes when you were in your thirties and to an hour or two in your forties. By the time you're in your sixties, you may have to wait an entire day or more after ejaculation before you can get hard again.

The amount of time you'll need to wait varies somewhat with the amount of excitement that you're feeling. Under very stimulating circumstances your refractory period may be shortened, and you may be able to respond more quickly.

Awareness of the changes that come with maturing is again the key here. If you try to get hard again too soon after ejaculation, you will naturally have difficulty getting a good erection. If you and your partner aren't expecting this, you may both feel a sense of anxiety, failure, and disappointment.

When you try again several days later, even though you've had an adequate rest period, worry about your previous failure can cause you to have trouble getting hard again. In other words, you can scare yourself into an episode of temporary impotence.

A very sensible way for you and your partner to avoid this kind of unpleasant outcome is to *accept* your body's message. If you can't get hard because it's too soon after your last ejaculation, don't try to force it. You can decide to wait for next time or you can choose to enjoy a very sensual lovemaking experience without an erection by caressing each other manually or orally. You can certainly use manual or oral stimulation to satisfy your partner and help her climax. Then, when your body is ready again for intercourse, you'll be able to go at it with a fresh spirit and enthusiasm.

Remember, too, that if you don't ejaculate you usually won't need a long rest period. So if your erection fades without a climax, you should be able to get hard again fairly quickly.

Other Changes   There are some other changes in the over-forty male that you may notice. For example, when you ejaculate, your semen will not be expelled with the same rocketlike force as when you were younger. The muscles behind the push aren't as strong as they used to be. This really shouldn't affect your enjoyment of your orgasms. After all, ejaculation isn't a distance contest.

When you were younger, you may have felt a sensation of impending ejaculation a few seconds before you actually climaxed. This is called the feeling of "ejaculatory inevitability," because you know that past that point you can't stop yourself from coming. As you've gotten older, you have probably noticed that this feeling seems to blend in more and more with the beginning of your orgasm.

You may also observe that after you climax your erection recedes more quickly than it did when you were younger. This is also one of the inevitable changes of aging, but one that needn't affect your enjoyment.

WHY THESE CHANGES OCCUR

Why these gradual changes as you pass forty? Why less need to ejaculate? Why more need for penile stimulation? Why slightly less hard erections?

The reasons are rather complicated. Erection, which you always experienced as a simple phenomenon—you saw your partner undressed, thought about sex, and your penis got hard—is actually a very complex process. It requires a precise interplay among various parts of your body. The first is your *brain*, as you respond to mental erotic stimulation and thoughts. The second is the erection reflex, which occurs when your penis is physically stimulated and impulses pass back and forth through your *nervous system*.

The nervous system acts by influencing a third mechanism,

a series of synchronized *vascular* actions. Your arterial system has to provide an adequate blood supply to your penis, while at the same time there has to be a partial blockage of the outflow of blood. This allows the blood to pool in special compartments in your penis and produces an effect like inflating a long, thin balloon. Your penis swells, becomes hard, and is ready for sex.

I'm about to describe what makes it all work. It's a little technical, but it is worth reading because it will help you to understand what can go wrong and what can be done to fix it.

The sexual stimulation, whether originally from erotic thoughts or from physical stimulation, causes impulses down certain nerves to the penis, where they cause the release of a chemical called *nitric oxide* in the smooth muscle of those compartments called the *corpora cavernosa*, which are going to fill up with blood to produce the erection. (When you get older, by the way, you keep the ability to respond to the physical stimulation reflex even after the mental stimulation reflex has weakened.)

The nitric oxide causes the release of another chemical called *cyclic GMP,* which causes the smooth muscle to relax and allows the blood to enter and fill up the corpora cavernosa, like filling up long balloons. As the arterial blood comes in with lots of oxygen, it produces lots more nitric oxide, which makes even more cyclic GMP. As those balloons fill they press on the veins that take blood out of the penis and compress them, trapping the blood and keeping the penis erect.

The penis then stays erect until the smooth muscle contracts again. Then the blood is forced out of the balloons and the veins are released as well and take the excess blood out of the penis.

The whole system is primed by adequate amounts of the male hormone testosterone, which helps control your erection mechanism and is largely responsible for sexual desire and arousal.

WHAT CAN GO WRONG

What I've described is how erection works ideally. The trouble is
that as you get older, this complicated system suffers some gradual wear and tear. Your reflex mechanism isn't as sharp. You may
develop some degree of high blood pressure and/or hardening of
the arteries (arteriosclerosis) in the vessels supplying blood to
your penis. This results in a decrease in its blood supply, less oxy-
genated blood coming in, and, consequently, a decreased speed
with which you can get hard.

The smooth muscle system that relaxes to allow the blood to
pool also developes arteriosclerotic thickenings or plaques and
may also not produce quite as much cyclic GMP. The result of
both of these changes is that the smooth muscle may not expand
as well as it did and the compartments may not fill up quite as well
as before. This in turn prevents them from fully compressing the
veins. You may therefore develop some microscopic leakage of the
pooled blood back out of your penis.

The result of all this is that erections take longer, require more
stimulation, are not quite as hard, go down more easily, and are
more fragile in general.

Another problem is that anxiety causes contraction of the
smooth muscle and lets the blood out of your penis. Therefore if
you start to worry about your erection, a self-defeating process
takes place. On the one hand, you stop having the sexual thoughts
that produce the nitric oxide. On the other, the anxiety itself
causes your erection to go down.

"Well," you might say, "don't be anxious." The trouble is that
when you know that your erection is more fragile, it's difficult not
to think about it. That awareness can turn into worry, and worry
can turn an otherwise fine erection into a limp one.

Finally, with every decade, your body's level of testosterone decreases. You produce less at thirty than at twenty, less at sixty than at fifty. This produces less frequent desire and less urgency for climax. There are probably other factors contributing as well, as simply increasing testosterone levels doesn't increase levels of libido back to young-adult levels. I'll discuss testosterone more fully in another chapter.

IN SUMMARY

As the erection system loses some of its sharpness of response, you'll start to notice the gradual changes in your erection that we've already described—slower erections, more need for stimulation, less firmness. But while your erection mechanism may have become more fragile and requires more help, keep in mind that for the most part *it's still working effectively* and should continue to do its job, right up through your sixties, your seventies, and beyond.

For a minority of men, however, the erection system gets derailed, and a real impotence problem, with inability to get erect, develops. Why does this occur?

To begin with, some older men have more severe breakdowns in their erection mechanism. Some have illnesses, such as diabetes, that can cause damage to the nerves responsible for the erection reflex. Others may suffer from pronounced hypertension, arteriosclerosis, or other conditions that may cause diminished blood supply to the penis. Diabetes can cause this as well.

Lack of testosterone may contribute to some men's problems. While the level of testosterone falls to some extent for every man, some men may develop a real deficiency.

Other extrinsic factors can unbalance an older man's more fragile erection mechanism—particularly alcohol, tobacco, and certain medicines, which we will describe at greater length in chapters of their own. Deficiencies of certain nutrients can play a part as well. Moreover, certain illnesses, pain, and—most important—anxiety and tension can all, individually or in combination, block your erection mechanism. These various factors that can potentially interfere with your erection prospects will be discussed more fully in subsequent chapters, along with ways you can maximize your chances for erection success.

WHY LOVEMAKING CAN BE BETTER AFTER FORTY

Many women have told me they feel that older men make better lovers. When they explain why, it's clear that the sexual changes of maturity contribute a great deal to what women like about making love with older men.

Barbara M., forty-two, told me, "It sometimes takes me a little while to get sexually excited. My first husband, who was my own age, was immediately erect and impatient for me to get turned on. My current lover, who is ten years older, takes some time to get ready, the way I do. We both stimulate and arouse each other, and for me that's a big plus.

"Bob usually needs me to play with his penis before he can get hard. I like being needed to produce his erection. It's nice to be able to help, and it makes me feel proud and excited when I make him hard. I enjoy the feeling of his penis getting firmer and firmer as I play with it. I feel that he's getting hard in response to me instead of just starting off that way.

"Lovemaking also lasts a lot longer. Young men seem ready to ejaculate right from the beginning, but Bob actually needs my help to climax at times. I can usually bring him to climax by making strong, active movements during intercourse. It's really fun watching him as I move.

"Every once in a while he has trouble climaxing at first. We just withdraw. Then I use my hands and my mouth to get him ready to climax and even lick his nipples while I'm playing with his penis, and then, when he's ready to come I insert him at the last minute.

"Either way, it makes me feel as if I'm giving him his climax, and that makes me feel like a skilled and sexy lover. I also really feel appreciated. The whole experience is more tender and sensitive and sensual and lasts longer. I think that all women like this."

As a younger man, the dominant theme in your sex life was the need to ejaculate. You became erect with little or no direct physical stimulation and were always in a hurry to proceed to intercourse. While you may have felt proud of this ability then, the pressure for rapid intercourse and rapid ejaculation doesn't fit the needs of most women, who usually take a little longer to get sexually excited. They may find younger men impatient, self-centered, and not willing to take the extra time needed to help a woman get aroused as well.

Women desire and appreciate more direct physical stimulation prior to intercourse and are generally more appreciative of lovemaking as a prolonged, sensual experience of which ejaculation is only a part. As an older man, you'll find that you will also enjoy the fullness of the lovemaking experience when you please your partner as well as yourself.

You are better prepared for the role in many ways now that you are older. You've had more experience and more time to learn how to best please your partner. You also have less need to push ahead toward a quick ejaculation. The now more gradual, sensual lovemaking focuses less on your penis alone and more on the whole mental and physical experience. Older men are better equipped, both mentally and physically, to please their partners as well as themselves.

Making love with an older man may be a more mutual love-making experience in other ways as well. A younger man's erection is simply there, and a woman may feel that she has had very little to do with the producing of it. But in making love with an older man, that same woman will most likely have a much more active role. She'll have the pleasure and personal experience of bringing about that erection herself, with her own two hands. It can give her a feeling of power, participation, and mutuality in your sexual relations that she very well may not have had before.

Often I've heard a woman say, as Barbara did, that she enjoys being needed in lovemaking. She feels proud when she can help her partner get hard and enjoys the feeling that he is becoming erect in direct response to her, and to what she is doing.

As an over-forty man coping with a variety of physical changes, you may feel that your need for penile stimulation represents a decline in your physical prowess. It is, however, simply a natural change, so don't overlook the great advantages in it for both of you.

You will, first of all, have the pleasure of your partner stimulating you in an endless variety of erotic ways. You'll also have the time and inclination to caress her at leisure, without being under internal pressure to hurry to ejaculate. And your partner will have the fun and enjoyment of exciting you, stimulating you, helping you to get hard, and perhaps helping you climax as well.

CHAPTER 2

THE VIAGRA REVOLUTION

I n the previous chapter we discussed the sexual changes that men experience as they age. These include needing less frequent ejaculation, requiring more stimulation and more time to get erect, having slightly less firm erections, and having erections that are more fragile and easier to disrupt. We then discussed the mechanism of how erections are formed and how things go wrong with age for that mechanism.

In this chapter we are going to discuss a remarkable medicine that works in a revolutionary way to overcome many of the erection problems that we've talked about. I'll explain how it achieves these extraordinary effects by working on the erection-producing mechanism that we discussed in the previous chapter.

First let me note that you may have heard some scary things in the media about Viagra, and about people who died while they were on this medicine. Much of the fear was greatly exaggerated, as it was pointed out that when you look at any group of millions of older men, with an average age in their sixties, some of them *will* die every year whether they take a medicine or not. There are dangers in using Viagra for certain people, especially people taking a certain class of medicines that I will explain to you, but keep an open mind. Viagra could change your life.

WHAT IS VIAGRA?

Viagra is an oral medication that comes in small, blue, diamond-shaped pills. The pill sizes are 25, 50, and 100 milligrams. To use Viagra, you take one pill, usually one-half to one hour prior to sex. Its peak effectiveness is usually about one hour, but it may work more quickly if you take it on an empty stomach and more slowly after a meal, especially after a high-fat meal. The medication often remains active for several hours after taking it.

WHAT WILL IT DO?

If you can already get erections, but they are not regular or secure, there is probably more than a 95 percent chance that Viagra will make your erections easier to obtain, firmer, and more difficult to lose. If you can't get erections, or get them very poorly now, there is probably at least a 70 percent chance that Viagra will be able to help you get erections that are adequate enough to function most of the time. (If you have not been able to have any erections at all for many years, you will probably require one of the other treatments that we will discuss later in the book.)

HOW DOES VIAGRA WORK?

Does all this seem too good to be true? Not once you understand how it works. Let me explain:

. You remember from our explanation in the previous chapter that erection occurs when smooth muscle relaxes in the walls of expanding compartments in the penis, allowing them to fill with blood. These compartments are called the corpora cavernosa. The blood is kept in the penis because these full chambers compress the veins leading out from the penis and thus trap the blood. This gives you the effect of a long, thin balloon that is blown up, full of fluid, and tied off at the outflow.

Again, what starts off the process and makes the smooth muscle relax? Sexual stimulation produces nerve impulses that cause the release of a chemical called nitric oxide in the smooth muscle. The nitric oxide activates another compound called cyclic GMP, which relaxes the muscle. This produces the erection. So that erections won't be permanent, there is an enzyme called PDE5 that breaks down the cyclic GMP and allows the erection to go down.

In the ordinary state of affairs, when you are having sex, sexual stimulation and arterial blood keep producing nitric oxide, which keeps activating cyclic GMP, while PDE5 keeps breaking it down. The buildup and breakdown stay in equilibrium, and you stay erect.

You will also remember that sexual problems arise because the smooth muscle in the corpora cavernosa doesn't relax well enough or the arterial vessels have enough arteriosclerotic blockage to slow down the blood from reaching your penis. If you are not clear on these details, it may be worth going back to the last chapter and rereading the explanation.

Now what does Viagra do in this cycle? Viagra inhibits the breakdown enzyme PDE5. This means that if you are sexually stimulated, the nitric oxide will keep producing cyclic GMP and it won't be getting broken down nearly as fast. Your erection will be easier to attain, firmer, longer lasting, and won't go down as readily. It's not magic—it follows clearly from the mechanism of erection that we have learned and the mechanism of the action of Viagra.

SIDE EFFECTS OF VIAGRA

Side effects of Viagra for the most part tend to be relatively mild. The most common are headache, flushing, dyspepsia (stomach discomfort), nasal congestion, and transient vision disturbances (usually a blue tint to the vision). They tend to be more frequent at the highest dose and less frequent at lower doses. The percentage of patients who discontinued Viagra in the test studies because of side effects was only 2.5. This is a very small number, and no more than those who discontinued while taking a placebo.

There is a *slight* risk of a condition called priapism, meaning getting an erection that won't go down. You might say, "How wonderful, an erection that won't go down!" but actually, after several hours, this could become serious because of the blood being trapped in the penis and the lack of circulation of new blood with oxygen. If you get an erection that lasts more than four hours you should call your doctor immediately or go to an emergency room to have the erection deflated.

People with sickle cell anemia, multiple myeloma, and leukemia are more in danger of having this side effect. If you don't have one of these conditions, priapism is an extremely unlikely side effect, especially if you stick with the recommended doses.

A REAL DANGER FOR PATIENTS TAKING
A CERTAIN KIND OF MEDICATION

As you now know, the nitric oxide released at the nerve endings causes a relaxation of the smooth muscle in the corpora cavernosa in the penis. Similar mechanisms work on the blood vessels elsewhere in the body. Nitroglycerine and other longer-acting nitrate medicines taken for angina take advantage of this, causing dilatation of the blood vessels in the heart (and elsewhere) by activating cyclic GMP, thus getting better circulation of blood to the muscles in the heart wall, and reducing angina.

You already know that Viagra blocks the breakdown enzyme for cyclic GMP in blood vessels in the penis. It also has the same effect in blood vessels throughout the body as well, but to a much, much lesser degree than in the penis. Ordinarily this causes no difficulty other than a slight, usually unnoticeable, drop in blood pressure.

However, if a patient takes nitroglycerine or a nitrate compound *along with* Viagra, the angina medicine causes the production of large amounts of cyclic GMP to dilate the blood vessels and relieve the angina, but the breakdown of this cyclic GMP is slowed by the Viagra. Even though Viagra's effect in these vessels is much less than its effect in the penis, the combination of Viagra with nitrates or nitroglycerine can cause a profound dilatation of the blood vessels, and therefore a severe drop in blood pressure. This can have serious, even fatal, effects.

It should be obvious that *patients on nitroglycerine or other nitrates cannot take Viagra*, and that this is not just an idle warning. It could mean your life! These nitrate medications have a number of different trade names, so check with your doctor AND with your pharmacist to make sure that you aren't taking them if you are going to start Viagra.

You may have heard about deaths of men taking Viagra. About four months after it became available, the media was sensationally reporting about seventy deaths in men who had taken Viagra. The FDA didn't get excited, though, because at that point several million men had been prescribed Viagra and the number of deaths *expected* from natural causes in a population of this many men with an average age of sixty would *actually be higher* than the reported number of deaths, even if the men weren't taking any medicine at all. As far as we can tell now, the only danger to life from Viagra is for men taking nitrates and for men whose hearts can't take the strain of sexual relations, with or without Viagra. We'll discuss sex with heart problems in another chapter.

INTERACTIONS WITH OTHER MEDICINES

Tagamet (cimetidine), a medicine for gastrointestinal distress, and all erythromycin drugs, which are antibiotics, will increase the concentration of Viagra in the blood. This means you probably will need a lower dose of Viagra if you are taking either of these kinds of drugs. Discuss this with your doctor.

VIAGRA FOR WOMEN?

Although Viagra is not yet approved by the FDA for the treatment of women, my discussions with researchers in the field indicate that it may have considerable benefit.

Preliminary evidence indicates that in posthysterectomy and

postmenopausal women who have suffered some loss of arousal and sensation and some diminution in ability to climax, Viagra can enhance sensation and arousal and make orgasm more intense. It seems to be effective in as many as two-thirds to three-quarters of these women. It apparently works, as in men, by bringing increased blood supply and relaxing the smooth musculature in the vaginal walls and the clitoris. This, in turn, causes engorgement of the vaginal walls and clitoris, which enhances sensation.

On the other hand, Viagra is unlikely to help a woman become psychologically aroused when personal emotional issues or unhappiness with one's partner is the core cause of the lack of arousal.

It seems to be more difficult to get approval for research on the treatment of women's sexual problems than for those of men because for men there is a clear visible impairment, easily measureable in an objective way: the penis either gets hard or it doesn't. For women the response is more subjective and less easily measured, and thus there is a tendency to say "Should we pay for this? What is the illness we're treating?" This has slowed down the research on Viagra in women, but as I have stated above, the early evidence is that it does work to help women as well as men respond sexually.

WHAT CAN VIAGRA MEAN
TO AN OVER-FORTY MAN?

Not everyone will want to try Viagra. Some people will prefer to perform "naturally." Others will be put off by the possible side effects. Still others may not be able to take it because they take nitroglycerine or other related nitrate compounds, or their heart condition may be unstable so that they may need nitrates without warning and their doctor doesn't want to risk the possible combination. (Viagra can increase the effect of nitroglycerine and nitrates, and the additive effect can cause a marked and quite serious drop in blood pressure—see above.)

For those couples who are willing and able to try this medicine, however, it can mean *no more worrying about erection!*

What does that mean? It means that if you are a man in his forties, fifties, sixties, or seventies . . . or even in his eighties, Viagra may be able to help you to overcome some of those normal changes of aging that we just got through telling you about in the previous chapter.

Let's assume that you are an ordinary, normal man over forty. You can get erections. You are not impotent. An understanding partner is a wonderful help, but for you, now, the overriding characteristic of your erections is that you have to worry about them.

Your erections are much more fragile than when you were younger. You may be able to get them sometimes and not other times, without apparent rhyme or reason. You and your partner may be reluctant to attempt sex sometimes because you can't always be sure you will succeed in getting erect. You may need more stimulation to get your erections, and when you do get them you may lose them more easily. It may require constant stimulation in order to keep your penis hard. If you are making love in the missionary position, for instance, and you'd like to move to another position, such as intercourse standing up leaning over the bed, you may be afraid to suggest it. You may be afraid that your erection will go down during the switchover and that you will then feel embarrassed and humiliated. The whole thing can feel embarrassing instead of romantic and pleasurable!

Consider what a medicine like Viagra could mean for you. As noted earlier, it comes in three sizes of pills: 25 milligrams, 50 milligrams, and 100 milligrams. The recommended starting dose for impotent men is 50 milligrams, and many impotent men need 100 milligrams. At 50 milligrams, and especially at 100 milligrams, Viagra may have significant side effects, such as stuffed nose, headache, foggy feeling, and blue-tinged vision, as described above. These only affect a small proportion of the men who use the medicine, but if they do affect you they can be uncomfortable and aggravating.

If you are a typical older man who is not impotent, however, but just has the type of fragile erections I just discussed, it's very likely you don't need 100 milligrams. You probably don't need 50 milligrams. Twenty-five milligrams, at most, or maybe even cutting a 25-milligram tablet in half (12.5 milligrams) will provide the security that you need, and it will do it with greatly reduced side effects. You still can't take it if you are taking nitroglycerine or other nitrates, but the minor discomforting side effects like stuffed nose and headache will be almost eliminated.

Remember that Viagra doesn't come in the 12.5-milligram size. It requires cutting the 25-milligram tablets in half, or cutting a 50-milligram tablet in quarters. You will have to experiment, under your doctor's supervision, to determine the correct dose of Viagra for you.

What will this low dose of Viagra do for you? Well, to summarize, your erections will no longer be fragile. You won't have to be reluctant to initiate sex for fear it won't work. If you can already get erections most of the time, this will be enough to guarantee that you will get hard almost all the time with adequate stimulation. And once you get hard you will stay hard, because Viagra prevents the breakdown of the chemical you produce in your penis in response to stimulation that makes you hard. Your erections should be firmer, which, although it probably won't matter to your partner, will make *you* feel better. You can change position, or walk around the room for that matter, and your erection won't go down. You will feel secure sexually. You will feel twenty years younger in bed.

When you ask your doctor for Viagra, he may tell you that you don't need it because you are not impotent. You will have to explain to to him or her that you understand that you are not impotent, but that you want to take it in low doses for security of erections. Ask him to read this chapter if necessary.

What won't Viagra change? Your desire, your need for sex, and your need for climax will still be less frequent than when you were younger. It will continue to take you a longer time to climax than when you were younger. You will still need to wait longer between ejaculations than when you were younger, and the volume of ejaculate will still be less. With Viagra you may be able to get erect a second time more quickly than without it, but it won't be the way it was when you were younger. Basically, as you can see, Viagra just helps with erections, but that is enough for most older men.

The real unrecognized benefit of Viagra is not just the way it can be used in the treatment of men with full-fledged impotence. It is what Viagra can mean for those much more numerous *ordinary older men* who are feeling insecure about their ability to function, and thus about their whole self-image.

WHAT WILL VIAGRA MEAN TO A WOMAN WHOSE PARTNER IS TAKING IT?

In the previous chapter we discussed some of the advantages for a woman in having an older male partner. They include having a partner who is not in such a hurry for quick intercourse and quick climax and who is happy with more and longer caressing prior to intercourse. The advantages also include having the fun and satisfaction of helping her partner get hard and climax, and generally having a more sensitive and sensual experience overall.

Some women worry that if their partners use Viagra they may lose some of these advantages and pleasures. There is absolutely no reason this has to be so!

If your partner is taking Viagra for erection security in the low doses we discussed, he will still need stimulation in order to get hard, although response will be easier for him, and even the visual stimulation of seeing you undressed may have an increased effect. He will not, however, have any increased urgency of ejaculation. He won't be in a hurry. He will still need just as much penile stimulation in order to climax as before. He should be glad to go slowly and to enjoy stimulating you and to have you stimulate him.

In fact, when your partner does get hard, he won't have to try to rush to insert his penis because of fear that he'll lose his erection if he doesn't enter. He *won't* lose it. And if he needed your help to climax before he started taking Viagra, he'll still need it.

Some women may worry that with Viagra their partners won't need them anymore. One woman whose partner was in his sixties said to me, "With Viagra he can have sex with anybody."

He always could have if he'd wanted to. If you have a good relationship, there's no reason he should now. One hears the occasional sensational story about a man who runs off after starting to take Viagra, but it only makes the newspapers because it is odd and unusual. Most relationships just improve, and women become every bit as happy with the improvements in sexual relationships as men.

If your female partner expresses this kind of concern, it's important not to laugh it off or treat it as a joke. It's time to listen seriously and reassure her that you love her and are not interested in anyone else.

WILL YOU LOSE SPONTANEITY?

As noted earlier, Viagra takes about thirty minutes to work on an empty stomach and probably close to an hour if you take it on a full stomach. If spontaneity means to you "Let's do it right now!" you will lose that. Of course, if you can do that without Viagra, you probably don't need the medication in the first place.

With Viagra, sex does require a certain minimum of discussion and planning: "Why don't you take your Viagra now and we can play around when we get back from our walk" or "Take the Viagra now and we can have a glass of wine and relax before we make love" or "I'll take the pill now and we can go to bed after I finish the dishes" or at the restaurant, "I'll take the Viagra with dessert and it will be ready to work by the time we get home."

Most people have an understanding about when they plan to make love most of the time anyway, so this really won't be that much of a change. Remember, you aren't on a fixed time schedule. The medication usually is effective for at least two hours from when you've taken it and perhaps even three hours, depending on circumstances. Pills cut open and taken on an empty stomach can work in as little as fifteen minutes. So, there is a lot of flexibility.

IN SUMMARY

Viagra is certainly not for everyone. Some people can't take it. Others just may not want to. They may feel it's not natural and that they want to function on their own and with their partners' help. If so, part 3 of this book, "Becoming A Better Lover After Forty," will be especially helpful to you. It deals with all the ways the two of you can use understanding, romance, ingenuity, and sexual techniques to improve your sexual lives.

On the other hand, some people may have both the ability and the desire to take a medication like Viagra to help overcome the variable sexual response that comes with getting a little older. If your erections have been fragile and not totally reliable, it may be worth talking to your doctor about whether a small dose of Viagra could change your life.

PART

2

SEXUAL CHANGES IN WOMEN OVER FORTY

CHAPTER 3

HOW WOMEN OVER FORTY CHANGE SEXUALLY

Women in their fifties, sixties, and seventies have occasionally come to me with what some might consider an unusual problem. These healthy, well-adjusted women were without sexual partners because they were divorced or widowed or because their husbands were chronically ill. What troubled each of them was that although she didn't have a sex partner, she continued to have strong sexual feelings that were difficult for her to deal with and control.

I remember Helen M. in particular, a woman in her midseventies, widowed, very active, working in her own small business. A new sexual relationship with a man seemed unlikely, but she found herself having frequent sexual fantasies and often feeling sexually aroused. Helen was afraid that she might, in her words, "do something foolish" and was distraught because she felt that

33

"a nice older woman" without a sexual partner wasn't supposed to feel sexual—and certainly wasn't supposed to be consumed with sexual fantasies and sexual feelings.

Helen was reassured to learn that it was normal for her to continue to have sexual feelings. She eventually formed a satisfying sexual and emotional relationship with an old acquaintance, a man seven years her junior who greatly appreciated her positive outlook about lovemaking.

Many people believe in the same old nonsense that Helen did—that women lose their sexuality as they age, especially after menopause. A few women do, in fact, experience a loss of sexual desire after menopause, and other women may use menopause as an excuse to end sexual lives that have been, for them, emotionally or physically unsatisfying. Most women, however, report no loss of sexual interest, sexual arousal, or sexual enjoyment after menopause.

SEX MAY BECOME MORE
PLEASURABLE AFTER MENOPAUSE

If you enjoyed sex before menopause and if you continue to have the opportunity for regular sexual activity, there is no reason why lovemaking shouldn't continue to be at least as satisfying for you as it was in earlier years.

The years after menopause may coincide with the departure of your children. This gives you and your partner more privacy for lovemaking and less of the feeling of constant fatigue that comes with caring for small children.

In addition, you might have been worried during your child-bearing years about becoming pregnant. Since menopause eliminates that possibility, it can mean increased sexual freedom for you.

Some women dislike having intercourse during their menstrual period or have discomfort with sex at this time. For these women, no longer having menstrual periods may be liberating and may mean expanded opportunities for comfortable, worry-free sexual relations.

After forty, women may also find that they're more relaxed about sex in general. During early years of sexual activity, many older women were still wrestling with their antisexual upbringings. They were often sexually inexperienced, hesitant to experiment, and unsure of how to please themselves or their partners.

For example, many women don't really learn how to climax until they've reached their thirties or forties. The discovery of orgasm is just the beginning of learning a wide range of techniques for enhancing lovemaking. As women become better at lovemaking and start enjoying it more, they tend to become much more uninhibited. They also tend to become more interested in learning about their sexuality. For these reasons, women over forty who are happy with their sexual partners often tend to find their sexual lives more satisfying than when they were younger.

As a woman over forty, you will likely be more sexually assured and secure and have more knowledge of your own physical responses. You've continued to improve your sexual skills, you've gradually shed sexual inhibitions over the years, and you've learned to identify your sexual needs and preferences. You may feel more secure about trying new techniques, such as oral stimulation, or new positions for intercourse. While at earlier times in your life you may have been reluctant to tell your partner what you like sexually, you are probably now more open and able to communicate. Nonetheless, you shouldn't ignore the fact that, as a woman over forty, you are undergoing certain physiological changes that may affect your sexuality.

YOUR HORMONE LEVEL FALLS
DRAMATICALLY AT MENOPAUSE

In previous chapters, we discussed how a man's body gradually undergoes physical changes and how these changes can affect his sexual response and desire. We also described how the hormone testosterone, which is the primary hormone responsible for sexual function in men, diminishes over the years. This slow decrease, as well as other imperceptible changes due to age, cause a man's sexual changes to be gradual, rather than sudden.

A woman, on the other hand, in addition to the slow changes of aging, experiences a dramatic, possibly jolting, decrease in her female sexual hormone, estrogen, at the time of menopause. The average age of natural menopause is about fifty, but the drop-off of estrogen levels is even more sudden if a woman has her ovaries removed at a younger age, for example during a hysterectomy. Unless her estrogen is replaced, a woman may have more abrupt physical changes in her sexual organs than a man has. On the other hand, because estrogen is not directly responsible for sexual desire, she usually won't experience the slowing of sexual response and desire that men do.

SEXUAL RESPONSIVENESS AND
SATISFACTION REMAIN CONSTANT

Testosterone, which in women is produced in the adrenal glands and ovaries, is responsible for sexual desire in both women and men. The few women who do experience a loss of sexual desire at the time of menopause can probably attribute it to a decrease in their supply of testosterone, rather than to a loss of estrogen. Lack of estrogen seems to cause diminished desire only when physical changes brought on by its absence cause sex to become uncomfortable.

Since a woman's physical sexual responsiveness is usually maintained after menopause, you should experience little change in your ability to become aroused or to achieve orgasm after menopause. Helen, whom we described at the beginning of this chapter, may have been somewhat unusual in the intensity of her sexual desire, but many women in their fifties, sixties, and seventies report that their sexual desire continues just as strong as it ever was. Older women often report sexual dreams, as well as multiple orgasms, during lovemaking. Moreover, many older women, even those at an advanced age, continue to masturbate if they are without a sexual partner.

ESTROGEN WITHDRAWAL AT MENOPAUSE

We all know that some women go through periods of extreme discomfort at the time of menopause. Symptoms can manifest themselves both emotionally (in anxiety, irritability, insomnia, nervousness, or depression) and physically (with hot flashes, fatigue, and headaches). All these are indications of *acute estrogen withdrawal:* of the body complaining about a marked drop in hormone levels.

These are not unusual symptoms, and you're not odd if you have them. Fully *85 percent* of all women have some hot flashes or other symptoms of acute estrogen withdrawal while going through menopause. About a fifth of these women suffer severely.

These estrogen withdrawal symptoms are simply your body's way of telling you it doesn't have enough estrogen.

It is commonly said that these symptoms can last anywhere from six months to as long as five years, but my gynecological consultants tell me that 25 percent of women still have some hot flashes *even after five years.*

There is no reason for any woman to have to undergo prolonged discomfort from estrogen withdrawal. These days, symptoms can be rapidly relieved by estrogen replacement therapy, which is usually readily prescribed for most women with acute menopausal distress.

LONG-TERM SEXUAL EFFECTS OF CHRONIC ESTROGEN DEPRIVATION

Hot flashes and the other signs of acute withdrawal are only the tip of the iceberg. Because menopause represents a permanent decrease in the amount of estrogen your body is producing, and because your body has stopped producing a large proportion of this important hormone, certain long-term effects will become evident *within five to ten years* after menopause.

The potential changes from chronic estrogen deprivation can be simply stated. Estrogen is specifically involved with the maintenance and development of your sexual organs, so a continued diminution in the supply of estrogen causes those organs to essentially atrophy, or shrink.

Thus, if you suffer a marked decrease in your estrogen level at menopause and you don't have estrogen replacement, you'll notice a gradual thinning of the walls of your vagina. When your ovaries were producing adequate estrogen, your vaginal walls were made up of thick, cushiony folds that allowed for a great deal of elasticity and expansion. It's this elasticity and ability to expand that allowed your vagina to accommodate a penis during intercourse and the passage of a baby during childbirth.

But the loss of estrogen following menopause causes a condition known as *atrophic vaginitis.* Your vaginal walls thin and become smooth, losing their soft folds and the cushioning effect that they previously had. The loss of elasticity may also cause narrowing of your vagina's opening, shortening of its length, and narrowing of its width.

Losing estrogen will also result in a loss of vaginal lubrication. Both the speed at which you lubricate and the amount of lubrication may decrease. When you were younger, your lubrication may have begun after just ten to thirty seconds of sexual stimulation. Now, it may take several minutes, and you may not get quite as wet.

The combination of these symptoms of chronic estrogen deprivation—loss of vaginal elasticity and cushioning, narrowing of the vaginal opening, and the decrease in lubrication—can make sexual intercourse uncomfortable. You may experience pain either on initial penetration or with deep thrusting by your partner.

Occasionally, older women who are not taking estrogen replacement also report urinary symptoms, such as burning, after intercourse. This is due to direct irritation of the urinary passage and bladder, since they are no longer as well cushioned or protected by the vaginal lining during intercourse.

A few women with severe estrogen depletion may experience painful uterine contractions during orgasm. These spasms can be eliminated with estrogen replacement.

Postmenopausal women also experience *thinning of the skin* in general and a loss of collagen and elasticity of the skin due to lack of estrogen.

Without estrogen replacement after menopause, most women

are likely to have some of the physical effects of decreased estrogen described above. Even so, their sexual interests and desires usually remain constant, and most women continue to enjoy a full sexual life.

On the other hand, a minority of women do report some loss of sexual desire following menopause. In some cases, the loss of desire is because sexual relations are uncomfortable due to lack of lubrication, narrowing of the vaginal opening, or other physical conditions. Other women may never really have enjoyed lovemaking (for more complex psychological or relationship reasons), and they use menopause as a convenient reason to discontinue it. Still others may find their partner unattractive or undesirable. Finally, for some women, as we mentioned above, diminished desire can result from lack of testosterone accompanying the loss of estrogen.

Another issue that makes some women give up on sex or lose desire is a feeling of embarrassment or self-consciousness about their self-image and appearance. Their bodies don't look the way they used to. They compare themselves to the young models portrayed in the media, and they are afraid that they no longer look attractive to their partners. Not feeling good about the way they look makes them not feel like making love.

Let me talk a little more about this issue of body image and appearance that upsets so many truly attractive older women, because it really is a shame and a distortion of reality.

Women are really bombarded with false images. Fashion magazines tend to portray anorexic, almost bizarrely thin models as the standard. Real women don't look like that. *Real women have curves*, not stick legs and bony chests.

On the other hand, magazines, catalogues, television, and other media tend to show luscious young girls in their late teens or early twenties. This can be very difficult for an older woman if you get conned into feeling that you have to compete with these young girls, that you have to look like them in order to be sexy.

Don't let the media do that to you! It will only bring unhappiness and dissatisfaction. It doesn't say anywhere that sex is reserved for girls in their teens and early twenties. If you think back to how unskilled and ignorant of sexual technique you were at that age, you will realize that you are now almost certainly a much better, and much more interesting, sex partner than those young girls would be.

SOME PHYSICAL ASPECTS OF SEXUALITY ARE UNLIKELY TO CHANGE

Not everything sexual changes at menopause. Although your breasts may lose some elasticity and may not swell as much during sexual arousal as they did when you were younger, your nipples will continue to become hard, erect, and sensitive with stimulation. If you enjoyed having your breasts caressed in the past, you should continue to do so after menopause.

Your clitoris will continue to respond to stimulation in much the same way it did prior to menopause. It will still become erect and firm, although because it may take somewhat longer to respond, you may desire more direct stimulation than you did earlier in your life.

Most women notice little if any change in their orgasms. Although laboratory measurements of uterine contractions during orgasm indicate that they may be somewhat less powerful and of shorter duration after menopause, most women report that they can't actually perceive any subjective change in their own climaxes.

NONSEXUAL BODILY CHANGES DUE TO
CHRONIC LACK OF ESTROGEN

We talked first about the *acute* estrogen withdrawal symptoms that primarily occur during the first five years after menopause. Then we discussed the *second stage* of chronic estrogen deprivation, the atrophy of the sexual organs that occurs about five to ten years after menopause. What I'm going to discuss now is the third stage, what many think of as *the disease process* of chronic estrogen lack. These conditions start to emerge after about ten years of estrogen deprivation and, unfortunately, are likely to affect women who do not, or can not, take estrogen replacement therapy.

Estrogen is a powerful hormone that has many natural functions throughout the body. Chronic estrogen lack can, therefore, bring on bodily changes that are not necessarily sexually oriented. Estrogen is intimately involved with maintaining bone calcification. Following menopause, many older women suffer from a marked acceleration of the loss of their bone calcium due to estrogen loss (as well as other factors such as decreased activity and decreased absorbtion of calcium). This may result in bones throughout the body becoming thin and fragile, resulting in a dangerous condition known as *osteoporosis.*

Severe osteoporosis can cause easy fractures of the hip, arm, or spinal vertebrae. This process of accelerated bone loss may be extremely prominent in women who have had an early menopause or have had their ovaries surgically removed earlier in life.

Osteoporosis isn't a minor or rare problem. We all know of older women who have fractured their hips and then been permanently incapacitated. Osteoporosis seems to be especially prevalent among women who are white and thinly built, who are heavy

smokers, who exercise little, who have poor lifelong calcium intake, and who have a family history of osteoporosis.

As many as 25 *percent* of white women over sixty may have
spinal compression fractures due to osteoporosis! Many older
women suffer from hip fractures that result in an acute deteriora-
tion of their level of functioning. Older women in the U.S. suffer
an almost unbelievable one and a half million fractures per year
due to osteoporosis.

It is also becoming clear that *arteriosclerosis and heart disease* are
probably accelerated by the absence of estrogen. Women who are
premenopausal seem to experience much less heart disease than
do men of the same age. But after menopause, when women are
no longer apparently "protected" by estrogen, their rates of arteriosclerosis and heart attacks tend to equal those of men.

After menopause, women's triglycerides and LDL (bad) cholesterol all rise, while HDL (good) cholesterol falls. All these negative changes are reversed by estrogen.

These effects on heart disease and arteriosclerosis are not trivial
or unimportant. Cardiovascular and heart disease are the primary
killers of women. Twice as many women die of cardiovascular and
heart disease as from all cancers combined! This includes breast
cancer!! Approximately ten times as many women die from heart
disease as die from breast cancer!!!

You can see why it's necessary to consider the risks of not taking estrogen replacement as carefully as the risks of taking it.

Although all women suffer a great deal of estrogen loss at
menopause, some experience much less than others because their
bodies continue to convert some of the weak androgens, made by
their adrenals, into estrogen compounds. Therefore, while all
postmenopausal women do experience some physical effects of
estrogen withdrawal, the degree varies widely. Probably as many as

50 percent of women suffer significantly, and 25 percent suffer severely, from this third-stage estrogen deprivation disease process if they don't have their estrogen replaced.

We'll look more closely at the role of estrogen in the next chapter.

CHAPTER 4

ESTROGEN REPLACEMENT AFTER MENOPAUSE

In spite of so many uncomfortable and even serious problems that can be caused by lack of estrogen, for many years estrogen replacement therapy wasn't universally recommended for all postmenopausal women. One reason, as I discussed earlier, is that, after the hot flashes subside, a lot of the most serious symptoms are things like cardiovascular disease and osteoporosis, which are relatively silent and not immediately apparent.

But a more important explanation is that estrogen is an active hormone and may have unwelcome side effects of its own, and until it became really clear, as it seems to be now, that the benefits of estrogen far outweigh the risks, women were sometimes unwilling to take it and doctors were sometimes reluctant to prescribe it. It is really only in recent years that large epidemiological studies are clearly establishing that the potentially more serious dangers lie not in taking estrogen but in going without it.

THE EARLY HISTORY

Before the 1940s and 1950s, menopause was conceived of as a natural and irreversible event. Symptoms of estrogen deficiency were simply considered inconveniences that older women had to endure. The most immediate discomforts of estrogen withdrawal, such as hot flashes, were treated with sedatives and exercise.

When estrogens became readily available five decades ago, doctors quickly realized that *estrogen replacement therapy (ERT)* would arrest the immediate symptoms of estrogen withdrawal such as hot flashes, but it soon became evident that ERT could also prevent other, long-term effects on the vagina and skeletal bones. It was not surprising that ERT rapidly became the standard therapy. By the 1960s, the hope was that women could "stay young forever" by taking estrogens.

THE UTERINE CANCER SCARE

Then, in the mid-1970s, the pendulum swung the other way. Reports of increased cancer of the uterus (endometrial cancer) among women taking ERT frightened many into stopping their estrogen therapy. This occurred despite the fact that uterine cancer is a very uncommon form of cancer, so that even with the indicated increase there was a very low incidence, and despite the additional fact that many, many more older women die each year from fractured hips due to osteoporosis—partly from estrogen deficiency—than ever die from uterine cancer.

Some women who had had hysterectomies even forgot that with no uterus they were in no danger from uterine cancer anyway. Doctors became very apprehensive about estrogen replacement therapy, and large numbers of women who might have been candidates for ERT were not treated with it. By the late 1970s, estrogen replacement therapy was generally used only if absolutely necessary, in the smallest dose and for the shortest time possible.

The medical community first hoped that estrogen creams could fill the gap and treat vaginal symptoms without exposing patients to the dangers of uterine cancer. These creams were applied topically to prevent vaginal shrinkage and dryness, but it soon became clear that the estrogen in the creams was rapidly absorbed. Using the creams resulted in blood levels of estrogen as risky as those caused by taking the hormone in pill form.

ESTROGEN/PROGESTERONE CYCLING

After much investigation into ERT, a number of researchers reasoned that perhaps the trouble was caused by administering estrogen steadily and without a break—or in giving it alone without progesterone, the other ovarian hormone that accompanies estrogen during the last two weeks of each menstrual cycle.

To explain why this should be so, we need a brief review of menstruation. In a normal menstrual cycle, estrogen stimulates the lining of the uterus (the endometrium) during the days before ovulation. Progesterone begins to be produced in significant amounts at the time of ovulation and accompanies estrogen until several days before menstruation. The combination of the two hormones in the latter part of the cycle produces an orderly buildup of cells to prepare the uterine lining for the possibility of pregnancy. At the end of the month, if no fertilized egg is implanted, the amounts of both hormones decrease sharply. The uterus then sheds its old, unused lining in the menstrual period and gets ready to start anew.

When menopausal women having ERT would receive daily doses of estrogen, without a break and without accompanying progesterone, it caused the lining of the uterus to be constantly stimulated and to grow in a disorderly fashion. Researchers believed it was this persistent stimulation and uneven cell growth that led to increased danger of uterine cancer.

Some doctors then began to recommend that their patients take estrogen only five days per week or else three weeks out of the month, in order to interrupt the constant stimulation. But the women's body fat stored the estrogen and released it during the days they weren't taking the hormone, so the uterus was still, in fact, receiving continuous estrogen stimulation. And it was estrogen alone, so the cells were still piling up in a disorderly way. Progesterone was what was needed to promote orderly growth, as well as monthly shedding.

Current evidence reveals that the uterine lining of postmenopausal women being cycled with a combination of estrogen and progesterone doesn't have the piling up of cells that comes from continuous estrogen stimulation; instead, it is normal in appearance.

In the early 1980s, a number of studies indicated that while postmenopausal women receiving estrogen alone had a higher rate of uterine cancer than did untreated postmenopausal women, those who received estrogen in combination with progesterone did not. In fact, women who took estrogen and progesterone cycled monthly actually turned out to have *fewer* cases of uterine cancer than did the untreated population.

This finding meant that estrogen replacement therapy with progesterone might even protect women from getting uterine cancer in addition to helping prevent osteoporosis (bone thinning), hip fractures, vaginal atrophy, and loss of vaginal lubrication.

ERT AND BREAST CANCER

When it became clear that cycled estrogen and progesterone seemed to eliminate the danger of cancer of the uterus, ERT became more widely used. A concern remained, however, that estrogen might increase risk of breast cancer. There were conflicting reports over a number of years, and some women remained reluctant.

The current status is that there are many studies with conflicting results: some showing an increased risk and some showing no increased risk. Usually when there is this kind of conflicting evidence, it means that if there is an increased risk, it is small.

It seems that if there is an increased risk, it is approximately the same as if your menopause had been delayed and you had continued to produce your own internal estrogen. It appears to be present primarily for women who have been on ERT for more than ten years. There is also some question as to whether any small apparent increase in risk is not really increased *risk,* but increased *detection,* as women on ERT tend to have more regular breast exams and mammograms than those who are not on ERT.

Since ERT is roughly equivalent to continuing on your own estrogen, it also means that you would continue to be protected from heart disease, bone thinning, and the entire disease process of estrogen deprivation which we discussed in the last chapter.

When one considers the overall risk/benefit ratio, there doesn't seem to be any question. Current medical opinion is clearly that Estrogen Replacement Therapy should be *standard treatment* for any woman who does not have a specific contraindication.

If a woman already has an "estrogen dependent" breast cancer (one that specifically grows in response to estrogen), obviouly she shouldn't take estrogen. However, interestingly, and almost incredibly, information is starting to emerge that a woman who is on ERT when she develops breast cancer has a better prognosis than a woman not taking ERT.

ERT AND CARDIOVASCULAR DISEASE

One of the many potential benefits of adequate estrogen levels is that the danger of heart attacks and arteriosclerosis may be reduced. Indeed, studies seem to show that postmenopausal women taking estrogen have a lower average annual death rate from all causes, but especially from cardiovascular disease, than do postmenopausal women who are not taking estrogen.

In other words, not taking estrogen increases your risk of dying, and especially increases your risk of dying from cardiovascular disease. As I explained in the previous chapter, this is not a small matter. Cardiovascular disease is the number-one killer of women, twice as common as all cancers put together. Increasing your risk by avoiding estrogen therapy entails a significant danger—much more danger, according to our current knowledge, than any danger from taking it.

Nothing about estrogen is entirely noncontroversial. Studies can be found that have shown conflicting results, but the prevailing medical opinion is that estrogen definitely offers significant protection when it comes to heart and vascular disease.

ERT CAN DECREASE OSTEOPOROSIS

As evidence accumulates, it is clearer and clearer that a major factor in the onset of osteoporosis in postmenopausal women is lack of estrogen rather than simple aging. Estrogen Replacement Therapy is the most effective single therapeutic agent in preventing osteoporosis in postmenopausal women. As we wrote in the last chapter, osteoporosis is a major, *major* problem. Twenty-five percent of older white women have compression fractures of the spine and there are more than one and a half million fractures per year in older women in the United States.

OTHER POSSIBLE BENEFITS

Emerging epidemiological studies indicate a number of other benefits from estrogen therapy that were not previously suspected:

- ERT seems to be protective against *colon cancer* with a remarkably large decrease in incidence.
- Estrogen seems to help women with *Alzheimer's disease,* although the improvement seems to be relatively small.
- Estrogen may protect against *adult macular degeneration* (a cause of blindness) and against *tooth loss.* And there are other possible benefits being investigated.

FEELING OF WELL-BEING

We've talked a lot about the medical and sexual benefits of taking estrogen, but there is another benefit that shouldn't be overlooked.

Women taking estrogen often just *feel* better. They have more of a sense of well-being and more ability to enjoy life. Estrogen seems to be simply life enhancing for older women, and that is not a small consideration. The average woman entering menopause has an expected life span of forty more years, and to be able to enjoy those years as much as possible is certainly a factor to weigh very importantly.

CURRENT MEDICAL OPINION ABOUT ERT

It appears that estrogen replacement therapy, when combined with progesterone, has become a new standard as treatment for postmenopausal women. The rewards and benefits seem to far outweigh the risks, on almost any scale of measurement.

As mentioned before, however, some women remain concerned about perceived dangers of estrogen replacement, while other intelligent women feel very conservatively that one shouldn't interfere with nature: if a woman's estrogen runs out when she's fifty-one, then so be it; the symptoms of estrogen deprivation are just a natural consequence of aging. "Why should I interfere with it."

Actually, though, chronic estrogen deprivation is a serious medical condition, with serious possible health consequences, which we have discussed at length. If you were seriously hypothyroid, to name another deficiency disease, would you say "I'll just live with it"?

You may not feel any immediate symptoms after you are past the hot flashes, but chronic estrogen deprivation is causing damage to your bones, blood vessels, and heart, to name a few organs. Don't ignore it because it's a "silent" disease, any more than you would ignore high blood pressure because you don't immediately feel sick from it.

Prevailing attitudes have changed before with new research and new studies, and they certainly could change again sometime in the future. Based on the best current evidence, though, it seems clear that ERT protects a woman from the sexual effects of chronic estrogen deprivation, and also protects her against osteoporosis and cardiovascular disease and perhaps other conditions as well, including colon cancer, tooth loss, and others. While there are some risks in taking ERT, the benefits seem to vastly outweigh them.

ADMINISTERING ESTROGEN/ PROGESTERONE CYCLING

Estrogen replacement therapy is now prescribed in a myriad of different regimens. Most contain Premarin (conjugated estrogen) or other estrogen compounds in combination with a progesterone hormone. They may be given in one of two different basic ways: They can be given continuously to avoid regular bleeding or, as an alternative, they can be given for about twenty-five to twenty-seven days, followed by three to five days with no medication to allow for shedding of the uterine wall (a short menstrual period). The estrogen and progesterone also come combined in a single tablet for convenience in Prempro for continuous administration and Premphase for cyclic. There are different possible doses of both the estrogen and the progesterone.

Estrogen also comes in vaginal creams (which are absorbed into the bloodstream), estrogen patches (and combined estrogen/ progesterone patches), and a new cervical ring delivery system. The possible ways you can take estrogen and progesterone are so varied and constantly changing that I won't attempt to recommend any particular way of taking it. Your choices are many, and you will need to discuss your choices with your doctor. Currently oral administration (taking pills) is still the most widely used, but that may change. In Europe the estrogen creams have become very popular.

If you've had a hysterectomy, you won't need the progesterone part and can take just the estrogen.

And finally, there is a new progesterone formulation just released, micronized progesterone (Prometrium), which is structurally identical to the progesterone your body produces and which seems to have fewer side effects than the synthetic progesterones that are still commonly used in this country.

Herbal formulations containing plant-source estrogens are generally not standardized in any meaningful way. Different brands, and even different batches of the same brand, may have vastly different potencies. There is no regulation. It may sound healthy to take "natural" estrogen, and it may give you a nice warm fuzzy feeling, but you have to consider whether this will be a *consistent, long-term* solution for a medical condition that you will be dealing with for thirty or forty years.

WHO SHOULDN'T TAKE ERT

As we have mentioned before, estrogen is not for everyone. Because it can exacerbate certain medical conditions, some women will have to avoid it altogether, while others will need to be closely monitored by their doctors. Check carefully with your personal physician to find out whether ERT is safe for you.

Any of the following conditions usually preclude a woman from taking ERT therapy:

- acute myocardial infarction (heart attack), although after recovery ERT may be protective against recurrences

- thrombophlebitis (blood clots)
- undiagnosed vaginal bleeding
- known estrogen-dependent malignancy such as breast cancer or endometrial cancer, or a *strong* family history (a sister or mother with breast cancer)
- pulmonary emboli (blood clots in the lungs)
- significant liver disease

Your doctor will also be particularly vigilant with ERT if you have migraine headaches, gall bladder disease, multiple sclerosis, high blood pressure, or seizure disorders (epilepsy)—all of which can be worsened by estrogens for some women, although estrogen can improve migraines, for instance, in others.

Caution must be exercised as well if a woman has endometriosis or fibrocystic disease of the breast. One's doctor is the person to evaluate these factors.

Any woman starting estrogen replacement therapy should have a thorough physical examination, including a breast and pelvic exam, a Pap smear, a blood pressure check, and possibly a chemistry profile.

You should have mammography every two years after age forty, and every year after fifty, whether you are taking ERT or not. (And if you have a strong family history of breast cancer, this should be moved up ten years.)

After receiving the green light from your physician and beginning estrogen replacement therapy, you may experience some bleeding each month, similar to a light menstrual period, if you are taking a regimen that causes this. This indicates a natural shedding of the uterine tissue, just as it was shed before your menopause. But be observant: if bleeding occurs when it shouldn't, during the days when you are not supposed to bleed, this may signal some uterine pathology, and you'll likely need an endometrial biopsy (a simple office procedure). See your physician immediately should this occur.

CAN I GET PREGNANT IF I USE ERT?

You may wonder whether pregnancy is possible when monthly bleeding resumes. The answer: If you're past menopause, you cannot get pregnant. Although the estrogen/progesterone cycling can produce normal uterine lining and monthly shedding, it cannot produce new eggs from your ovary.

OTHER OPTIONS BESIDES ERT FOR MAINTAINING SEXUAL ENJOYMENT

Many alternatives are available to help keep your lovemaking enjoyable and your vagina healthy, whether or not you choose to take estrogen replacement therapy.

To begin with, maintain an active sexual life, if possible. Masters and Johnson have reported that women in their sixties and seventies who continue to have sexual contact once or twice a week continue to lubricate quickly and well. These women also continue to have good vaginal expansion during intercourse in spite of their age, their lack of estrogen, and the thinning of their vaginal walls.

There may be a time in your life when your partner is not available or when you don't have a partner. If so, one way to keep physically toned and sexually responsive until you do have a partner again is by masturbating. Postmenopausal women who are unable to have sexual relations but don't remain physically active through masturbation may experience some narrowing of the vaginal opening and shortening of the vaginal canal. As a result, they may have some temporary discomfort when they resume sexual relations in the future.

Some women occasionally insert a penis-sized object in their vaginas during masturbation. Appropriately shaped dildos or vibrators are available in sexually oriented shops, through mail-order catalogues, on the Internet, and through some sexually oriented magazines.

One of my patients, Harriet M., shyly told me that she was embarrassed to buy a vibrator, so she simply used a cucumber or squash. She said they were just the right shape, were inexpensive and readily available, and had no sharp edges. She smilingly said that the only problem she had was blushing at the grocery store checkout counter.

Of course, anything you insert in your vagina should be clean, and long enough so that you can extract it easily.

Another way to keep yourself in shape is to tone your pelvic muscles by doing Kegel exercises, which are recommended after childbirth to reestablish vaginal tone, but which you can also use to keep your own vaginal tone healthy. These exercises are easy and can be done almost anywhere. They'll be described at greater length in chapter 14.

Vaginal lubricants. If you find that your vaginal lubrication is diminished, lubricants can greatly help to prevent painful intercourse, as well as irritation of the urinary passages following intercourse. There is a great variety of choices.

Petroleum jelly (in the form of Vaseline) is fairly widely used. I recommend against its use, however, since it's not water soluble and can clog your pores and urinary passage.

K-Y Jelly is an all-purpose sterile medical lubricant and is odorless and clear and safe to use.

Other vaginal lubricants are made especially for lovemaking.

One interesting one is Kama Sutra Oil of Love, which is scented, tastes good, and imparts a warming feeling when you rub it or blow on it. It's available on-line and in specialty shops.

One of the best products specifically designed to be a vaginal lubricant and to be used during sex is a product called Astroglide. It's available in many pharmacies. Unscented and colorless, it washes off easily and it won't stain. It won't provide the sensuality a flavored lovemaking oil like Kama Sutra will, but it has the consistency of natural vaginal lubrication. As a simple vaginal lubricant it's quite effective, and I do recommend it.

There are other similar products; if you can't find Astroglide, just ask your pharmacist to recommend another lubricant.

In an emergency, a vegetable oil from your pantry will be smooth and provide good lubrication. An oil such as olive or corn oil, for instance, is edible and thus won't detract from oral sex. And it has no cholesterol. One disadvantage: Vegetable oils can stain the bedsheets.

Finally, one highly inventive patient told me that she uses the juice of an aloe vera leaf as a vaginal lubricant, and that she and her partner are very happy with it.

OTHER OPTIONS BESIDES ERT TO HELP PREVENT OSTEOPOROSIS

It seems clear that estrogen is the strongest factor in preventing osteoporosis. However, some women can't take estrogen. If you are one of these women and are unable to take estrogen because of medical problems, there are other ways in which you can help prevent osteoporosis.

Of course, as well as being stimulative to bone growth, estrogen is also stimulative to the sexual organs and breasts, as we have discussed. While these effects are beneficial for most women, for some, such as those with an estrogen-sensitive cancer, this stimulation can be dangerous.

This has led to a search for designer estrogens, which would have some of the effects of estrogen but not others. This new class of medications is called Selective Estrogen Receptor Modulators (SERMs), because they have only some selected actions out of all the actions that regular estrogen has.

Evista (raloxifene), the first of this new class of medications, has recently been released. Evista activates the estrogen receptors in bone, but not the estrogen receptors in the breast, which makes it a safe way for women to prevent osteoporosis even if they can't take estrogen. The disadvantages are that it competes with any existing estrogen so that it increases hot flashes and doesn't prevent vaginal atrophy. It also may not protect against heart disease the way estrogen does.

Tamoxifen, another SERM, also protects bone density without any breast cancer risk. However, like Evista, it increases hot flashes. It also actually worsens vaginal atrophy. Tamoxifen does not give an estrogenlike protection against heart disease, and there is an increased risk of endometrial cancer.

Aside from these new medications, there are other practical actions you can take to help protect yourself against bone loss. Adequate lifelong *calcium* intake is very important. Calcium supplementation during the postmenopausal years can also help you slow down or avoid loss.

The addition of *vitamin D* (400–800 units/day) and fluoride to a postmenopausal woman's diet has been shown to be effective in retarding the progression of osteoporosis once it has been diagnosed. These should be taken, however, only under the direct supervision of a physician to avoid overdosage. (Excessive vitamin D, for instance, can cause kidney stones.)

One of the most important things you can do to maintain your bone structure and prevent osteoporosis is to get adequate amounts of moderate exercise such as walking, jogging, etc. Exercising with weights, even small amounts of weight, also helps maintain bone density. Inactivity contributes greatly to loss of bone substance. Again, the best advice on how much exercise will be good for you will come from your own personal physician.

Fosamax (alendronate) is a medication that, in combination with calcium and vitamin D, increases the density of bones by inhibiting bone resorbtion.

Finally, *smoking* highly correlates with bone thinning. Need I say more?

PART

3

BECOMING A BETTER LOVER AFTER FORTY

CHAPTER 5

OVERCOMING ERRONEOUS EXPECTATIONS ABOUT MALE SEXUALITY

One of the paradoxes of an older man's life is that he can order nearly every part of his body to do his will—but his penis, whose behavior is so important for his self-esteem, seems out of his control and often behaves in ways that are very frustrating for him. In fact, the more he anxiously tries to control it, the more trouble he's likely to have.

He can't get his penis erect by sheer will. He has to wait for the appropriate stimulation to make it happen. The more he worries or tries to get hard, the less likely he is to succeed. He feels embarrassed and humiliated if he doesn't get erect when he thinks he should, and he fears being a failure in his partner's eyes.

Men over forty, therefore, often have great concern about their sexual lives and a great deal of anxiety about their sexual performance. They often believe they have to live up to unrealistic expectations about male sexual performance—expectations that a "real man" can have an erection whenever he wishes, unassisted and without help, that his erections are always full and firm, that he constantly feels ready for sex, and that he can make love to his partner anytime she desires. These expectations are difficult to live up to at any age, but after forty, most men can't even come close to such unrealistic goals.

In my practice treating impotence and other sexual dysfunctions, I saw a great many older men, and I was constantly struck by how many of them were plagued by these same unrealistic expectations and by how these expectations contributed to their sexual problems.

I remember George M., sixty-five, who told me that his wife wouldn't touch his penis because she was "an old-fashioned woman." His goal was to get unassisted erections from caressing her "the way I always did." I had to tell him that those days were gone forever, but that if his wife realized that *he needed her help*, she probably would be glad to assist (she was), and that they would then both enjoy lovemaking more than ever (as they did).

Sometimes unrealistic expectations create sexual problems where there really weren't any to start with. Men begin to worry so much about not living up to those expectations that the worry, in itself, causes genuine sexual dysfunction. A man with enough anxiety about his performance may end up actually unable to get erect, unable to maintain his erection, or ejaculating too rapidly because he is hurrying to use his erection before he loses it.

Patients frequently come to me with one or more of the following five complaints, which often turn out to have their origin in erroneous expectations.

"I'M NOT GETTING ERECTIONS ANYMORE"

Too many older men tell me they're not getting erections anymore and have even stopped having sexual relations, when there is really nothing wrong with them at all! What they mean when they say they're not getting erect is that they are no longer experiencing the frequent, unassisted erections they got years ago.

Now that you're over forty, sooner or later you're going to require more direct physical stimulation of your penis in order to get hard. This doesn't happen to all men at the same age, but as you get older you'll certainly find that spontaneous erections happen less and less frequently. If you and your wife keep waiting for that spontaneous erection to occur before starting sex, you may eventually find yourself waiting a month or more.

Having your partner help you get hard is natural and normal and, besides, it can be fun for both of you. Your erections may not be spontaneous anymore, but your lovemaking can be as spontaneous as you like. You can make love whenever the mood strikes the two of you, as long as your partner is willing to help.

"MY ERECTIONS AREN'T ROCK HARD THE WAY THEY USED TO BE"

That's right, they probably aren't. Your erections at age forty, fifty, sixty, or seventy will probably not be as hard as they were when you were eighteen. So what! As long as they're hard enough for enjoyable lovemaking, they can give you and your partner all the pleasure you want.

You're probably a much more skilled lovemaker now than you were at twenty, and you are probably much more effective at pleasing a woman now than you ever were then, even though your erections may have been harder in those days.

Many men have the erroneous belief that their proficiency as lovers is in direct proportion to the hardness of their erections. Worrying about how hard your erection is will only serve to interfere with your excitement—and that will just make the erection softer. So stop measuring the hardness of your erection and just go ahead and enjoy it.

"I CAN'T HOLD MY ERECTIONS"

Many men I treat believe that they're entitled to only one erection per sexual encounter. They feel that one erection has to last the entire lovemaking time—be it five minutes or forty-five—and that once it's lost it's gone for good.

There's no reason this should be so at all. Where is it written that you're allowed to have only one erection? During the course of extended foreplay your erection may come and go three or four different times, even if you stay mentally very sexually excited and desirous. There's nothing wrong if this happens. It's perfectly natural. So if you have an erection and lose it, either prior to entry or even during intercourse, there's no reason for panic and no reason to feel ashamed. Just ask your partner to help you get your erection back, or stimulate her orally or manually until your erection returns. She'll appreciate the extra lovemaking as much as you do.

If you're getting firm erections, losing them during lovemaking becomes a problem only if it happens whenever you attempt to penetrate, thus preventing you from enjoying intercourse at all. This probably means that the problem is being caused by anxiety about your performance.

If you are consistently losing your erections and this is seriously interfering with your sexual relations, it might be worth trying low-dose Viagra as described in chapter 2, "The Viagra Revolution." If the problem is physical, this may help. If the problem is anxiety, the Viagra will help for sure, and after using it one or two times, just having it in reserve my give you enough confidence that you may stop worrying and be able to keep your erections without further use of the medication.

Another way to deal with the loss of erections is the Teasing Technique, as we will explore in chapter 9, "How to Help Your Man Get Firm Erections." The Teasing Technique is a sexual exercise that you and your partner can use together to help you overcome the problem in a natural way.

"SOMETIMES WHEN WE HAVE SEX I CAN'T EJACULATE"

It's surprising how many men worry that they have a serious sexual problem because they occasionally can't reach a climax. When this has happened, what they've often done has been to attempt to force the climax, working harder and harder at it, until they become frustrated, scared, and lose their erections.

Most older men discover that even though they may be fully aroused and excited, they don't have the need to climax every time they have sex. They learn to accept this as a normal part of their lovemaking. It doesn't interfere with their enjoyment, and it isn't a problem to them unless they think of it as one.

If you're tired, under stress, or have had a climax fairly recently, you may not feel the need to climax. In fact, you may not even be able to climax. This is simply your body's way of telling you that it doesn't need an orgasm at that moment. Trying to force it will only get you into trouble.

If you just relax and enjoy your lovemaking and don't worry about whether you climax or not, you'll find that you may be able to continue with intercourse for a long time (to your partner's great pleasure). And, since you don't really need a climax, missing it won't cause you to feel sexually frustrated afterward.

In fact, if you don't climax, you may keep your feeling of sexual stimulation so that you'll be able to have sex again later the same day. You won't have to wait as long as you ordinarily would before your sexual desire returns.

"I'M NOT ALWAYS READY FOR SEX
THE WAY I USED TO BE"

One of the myths that can get you into trouble is the one that claims a man should always be interested in having sex, and that he should always be able to get aroused as long as he has a willing and attractive partner.

We certainly don't expect that kind of response from a woman. While some men may inconsiderately expect their partners to be ready for sex at any time, most men and women realize that a woman usually needs a favorable emotional and physical environment in order to be sexually responsive and to become sexually aroused. She'll respond more readily, for instance, if she's in a relaxed frame of mind than if she's feeling stressed, tired, or worried.

Men, on the other hand, seem to feel that they should get turned on anytime their partner expresses willingness or interest. They may even be ashamed and embarrassed if they don't, or feel they are not fulfilling their masculine duty. This is very unrealistic, especially for men over forty.

As your need for climax gradually decreases in frequency, you will also discover that there are times when you're just not very sexually responsive—whether it's because you're worried or tired or just not feeling sexy, or for no particular reason. If this occurs, you may sometimes be able to get turned on with enough encouragement, but at other times it just may not be in the cards. If this occurs, there's no reason for concern. Just help your partner climax manually or orally if she's already excited, and wait until the next time for yourself.

IN SUMMARY

A lot of a man's feelings about how successful he is as a person depend on how successful he sees himself sexually. And most men, even those who really know better, have a nagging residue of some of these myths. Their unrealistic expectations, along with those of their partners, can produce much unnecessary heartache.

If this describes you as a couple, you may be able to really open up your sexual lives by relaxing your preconceptions about exactly how lovemaking should be, thus enjoying a wider variety of sexual experience. The years after forty, when both of you have more leisure to explore sexually, are ideal for this.

CHAPTER 6

OVERCOMING MENTAL OBSTACLES TO REALLY GOOD SEX

My practice taught me that there are many men and women over forty who would really like to enjoy sex more, but who find that some of their own ideas and thoughts block their enjoyment. They envy other men and women who appear to have free and open pleasure in their sexual lives, and they fear they may never be able to achieve it for themselves.

But it doesn't have to be this way. You can learn to be free sexually. You can learn to let yourself go, bypass distracting thoughts, reevaluate and shed old inhibitions, and change your preconceived ideas about lovemaking.

OVERCOMING THOUGHTS THAT CAN DISTRACT YOU FROM FULLY ENJOYING LOVEMAKING

Has the ability to enjoy, really enjoy, your lovemaking frequently been blocked by distracting thoughts that interfere, worry you, or undermine your arousal? Such thoughts can spoil an otherwise enjoyable lovemaking experience by preventing you from getting into a lovemaking mood or by ruining one after you're in it. They can block your excitement and prevent you from getting erect if you are a man; they can prevent you from becoming aroused, from lubricating, or from climaxing if you are a woman.

Each of us has experienced such mental interruptions at one time or another. But there are ways around them.

Simple distractions can cause your mind to drift away from sensual feelings of lovemaking. They can lead to thoughts like

It's too hot (or cold) in here.
Are we making too much noise? Can anyone hear?
I think I need to go to the bathroom.
My arm is sore.
I wish the faucet would quit dripping.
What should we have for dinner?
What if the kids come home?
I have to get that report out tomorrow.

Insecurity thoughts, especially worries about your own attractiveness, can make you preoccupied with your appearance or desirability instead of enjoying your partner's caresses:

My skin looks flabby.
I'm getting a potbelly.
I didn't shave my legs.
I wonder if I look fat.
He (or she) probably doesn't really enjoy caressing me.
I wonder if I smell bad.

Concern about your sexual performance can also get in the way of
your enjoyment of sex and may even block successful functioning:

I don't think I'm going to get hard.
I wonder if I'm wet enough.
I don't think I can climax.
My penis isn't hard enough.
I'm taking too long to come.
He (or she) is probably getting tired of caressing me.

Worries about erection can often be self-fulfilling, with the resulting anxiety crowding out all your sensual feeling and actually
preventing you from getting hard.

The same is true for women when it comes to arousal or climax. If your mind is filled with worries that you aren't getting excited or that you won't climax, those worries can bring about
exactly what you fear.

Putting sex last in your priorities can become a major problem.
Many people feel that they don't have time for sex. You may not
think of it in exactly those terms, but you may always feel that
there is something else "more important" that you should be doing. This may be because you haven't really been enjoying lovemaking or because you have been raised to feel that sex (and other
pleasures) shouldn't be important to you or to your partner—especially now that you are older. In either case, the result is that

lovemaking is given a low priority in your life. This can lead to such distracting thoughts about time priorities during your lovemaking as these:

I don't have time for this.
I should be doing the laundry (or working on next week's proposal, or whatever).
I'm not going to get enough sleep.
Let's get it over with as fast as possible.

Holding on to irritations and resentments can be particularly destructive to your sexual enjoyment. Here we have:

I'm still angry at him (or her) for what happened earlier (or yesterday, or last week, or eight years ago).
I'm just having sex because he (or she) wants it.
He (or she) only acts nice and gives me attention when there's going to be sex.

Worry about other problems having to do with your business, your children, money, or what you need to do tomorrow can make it very difficult for you to fully engage in satisfying lovemaking.

STEPS TO A SOLUTION

How can you overcome these blocks to your own enjoyment? The first step is to decide, and then make absolutely clear to yourself, that you *DO WANT* to enjoy lovemaking—for you, yourself. You may also want to take part in lovemaking for your partner's pleasure, but it's important to be clear in your own mind that having the pleasure, intimacy, and satisfaction of good lovemaking is something you desire, and that you don't want to spoil the experience with worry and resentments. Making this decision is an important, even crucial, step toward successful lovemaking.

Reconsider Priorities   During the course of an ordinary day, you constantly order your own priorities, choosing to do certain things in place of others that would also be possible. It's important to choose lovemaking as a high priority in your list—more important than doing household chores or working on next month's financial report. The pleasure, warmth, and intimacy that you will get from satisfying lovemaking will mean more to you the next day, much more than getting an extra half hour or forty-five minutes of sleep. It really will!

Put Aside Resentments   If you are troubled by feelings of irritation and anger during lovemaking, you've probably found that it's difficult to set aside some of the hurts from the past as well as fresh arguments and disagreements. Indeed, some hurts are too big and too painful to overlook; only you can decide that. Realize, however, that holding on to your anger and resentment during lovemaking strongly interferes with your ability to respond sexually and to enjoy your lovemaking.

Perhaps it would help to keep your *LONG-RANGE* goals in mind. Are you aiming for a relationship tomorrow, next week, or next month, in which you and your partner are still angry and unhappy with each other? Or would you like your relationship to be one in which you are sharing, intimate, and loving? If you really want this second kind of relationship, try to put aside your resentments while you are in bed. You'll have plenty of time to take them up in a neutral atmosphere later, if they still seem significant. Good lovemaking has a wonderful, healing effect. Sometimes the petty irritations that were so important before lovemaking seem inconsequential after you've enjoyed a happy sexual experience.

Focus Your Thoughts on Your Actual Physical Sensations
Some useful techniques can help you control the distractions, worry, and thoughts of insecurity that wander into your mind and get in the way of your sexual response.

The most simple, yet direct, method is to focus your thoughts on the physical sensations you are receiving. Instead of dwelling on the roof needing repairs or worrying that you are not getting excited fast enough, focus on your actual physical feelings. Consider the feeling of smoothness, softness, or warmth of your partner's touch; the feel of that skin against yours, the warmth or roughness or coolness; if you are a man, the tingling feeling in your penis as your partner slides her hand up and down its shaft; if you are a woman, the feelings in your nipples, clitoris, or vagina. Relaxing and concentrating on these things will help establish your own sensual mood.

Tell Each Other About Your Feelings and Sensations You can carry this technique one step further by relating what you are feeling, or by having your partner describe his or her sensations to you. This can be very sexually arousing as well as helpful in focusing your thoughts.

You might say, "Your hands feel really smooth and soft on my back," or "Your vagina feels really hot and wet around my penis." Or your partner might say, "Your tongue feels wet and velvety on my nipples," or "Your penis feels like it's filling up every bit of me." This type of passionate, sexually explicit dialogue can rapidly banish irrelevant thoughts.

Fantasize   Fantasy can be a very powerful way of focusing your thoughts on the sensual. Try imagining yourself in an especially sexy scene. You can fantasize about a previous encounter, about sex in a particular position or circumstance, or about how you would like to make love then and there. Or you can recall feelings you had in some particularly romantic or exciting lovemaking episode.

It can also be arousing to fantasize about what the lovemaking feels like to your partner, and to imagine yourself in his or her place. For example, if you are a woman, imagine how exciting it must feel for your partner to have his penis sliding in and out of your vagina and to feel its velvety, warm wetness. If you are a man, imagine the sensations that your partner must have as she feels your penis inside her, filling her up. Sharing your partner's feelings like this will give you a whole new perspective.

Help Each Other Overcome Distractions   If you are having trouble focusing or concentrating on lovemaking, learn to tell your partner and ask for his or her help. If you explain, for instance, that you can't concentrate because you're worried about some irrelevant concern, your partner may be able to help by talking sexily to you, by describing his or her sensations, or even by reassuring you.

Similarly, you can help your partner by giving positive feedback and reassurance. A woman whose partner has been worrying about his erections, for example, might say as she begins to feel him becoming aroused, "I can feel you getting excited—you're getting firm and warm right in my hands."

If you are a man and your partner is having trouble concentrating, you can describe the feeling of her nipples getting erect, her clitoris rolling under your finger, or the wetness and firmness of her vagina gripping your fingers or penis.

Sometimes, if your partner is preoccupied or worried, making him or her laugh can be another very effective way to break the worry cycle and produce a more relaxed state.

Remember that you can control distracting and interfering thoughts. It's most important to make up your mind that you *DO* want to enjoy lovemaking; you *DON'T* want to be blocked by resentments, by minor aggravations, or by worries; and that you are going to give lovemaking a high priority in your life.

OVERCOMING THE INHIBITIONS THAT PREVENT YOU FROM BEING FREE

The leftover inhibitions from our antisexual upbringings can also get in the way of our full enjoyment of sex. These include all too many irrational rules about what's right and proper—making love at the "right" time and in the "right" place and in the "right" way. Worrying about everything being right and proper can, unfortunately, really limit your sexual horizons, give you a negative attitude about lovemaking in general, and be very damaging to your loving relationships.

Imagine that you're in the bathroom shaving. Your wife comes up behind you and rubs your chest and then slides her hand down and brushes it over your penis. Are you likely to say something like "I'm busy now"?

If you are a woman and you are in the middle of putting on your makeup and your husband comes up and gently squeezes your breasts, are you likely to say the same thing?

Stop and think: What does "busy" have to do with it anyway? How long will a penis caress or a breast squeeze take? Certainly no more than fifteen or thirty seconds. It won't hurt your shaving or your makeup to take a thirty-second break.

I think the concern that prevents many people from enjoying this kind of play is the feeling that the sexual touching will inevitably lead to intercourse. There's no reason that it has to do so at all. If your partner caresses you while you're shaving, you could turn around and give her a hug and even rub her vaginal area with your hand, tell her how good her touches feel—and then go back and finish your shaving. She'll feel wonderfully rewarded for her efforts, and you'll both have a nice glow.

You may decide sometimes to stop whatever you're doing and go ahead and make love right then and there on the bathroom counter, but it's certainly not required. You can exchange sexual touches and caresses in the same way that you give hugs, as a way of expressing your affection for each other and of telling each other that you're desirable and desired. Accepting a sexual caress with appreciation and enthusiasm doesn't commit you to intercourse.

It's the same if the two of you are in bed at the end of a long day and your husband leans over and licks one of your nipples. You could turn away with a lot of negative body language and remind him how tired you are, or on the other hand, you could tell him that the other nipple needs a lick too. You could then give him a big hug and tell him how much you appreciated his licks but that you're really exhausted and ready for sleep.

What a difference there'll be in the way the two of you go to sleep! The first response is likely to project a feeling of annoyance and being pressured on your part and produce a feeling of being rejected and hurt on your partner's. The second response may well allow you both to feel appreciated, content, and loved. And who knows—you may even decide you aren't as tired as you thought and go ahead and enjoy lovemaking anyway, even if it's just a little appetizer of the kind described in chapter 13, "Prolonging Your Lovemaking for Hours."

If your partner suggests making love leaning over the bathroom counter or the bed or sitting in a chair, do you find yourself reacting with an immediate negative response without even thinking? Do you tend to feel that making love in different positions or in different ways is somehow "not nice" or even perverted?

Stop and think! Why in the world should the position that you're lying or standing in when the penis goes into the vagina have anything to do with rightness or wrongness or with morality in any way? Don't restrict your lovemaking unnecessarily. Allow yourself the adventure. Experiment with all the myriad positions and types of lovemaking that you and your partner might enjoy.

If you've just finished a leisurely Sunday breakfast alone together and your partner slips her hand inside your pajamas, are you likely to take her hand away and say "not here" or "not now"? But why not here? And why not now? Why should it be that sexual touching is allowed only in one room of your house, the bedroom? Whoever said that sexual touching was appropriate at night in bed but not in the morning after breakfast? Yet many of us harbor such leftover feelings of what's proper and what's not.

When you find yourself starting to get these "not here, not now" feelings, try to examine them yourself. Is there anything really wrong with right here and right now? Sexual touching or even making love in unexpected places and times can kindle a new feeling of sexual interest and inspire vitality in your lovemaking. It can add variety and excitement and a feeling of being deliciously daring.

Try to get away from all those concerns and negative messages about sex. Quit worrying about what your mother or your friends would think if they knew that you were making love in broad daylight right here on the dining room table. Your mother's not here. When and where it's appropriate for you and your partner to make love privately is your own decision—whether it's in the morning, in the dining room, or on the sofa, if you so desire.

Leave yourselves open to experiment and allow yourself to give or receive sexual touches at any time without feeling annoyed or irritated. Getting your mental obstacles out of the way will keep you from depriving yourself of pleasure, warmth, and feelings of being loved.

CHAPTER 7

SEXUAL VARIETY

Romance and Sensual Adventures

For too many older couples, lovemaking has lost its spontaneity. They find themselves always making love in the same way, in the same place, at the same time. It's usually in bed, in the dark, before going to sleep, and with no romantic atmosphere whatsoever.

If this is the way your lovemaking is going, you may be justified in feeling that it's becoming dull and boring. When you think of making love in romantic settings, it may sound to you as if it's fine for someone else but not something you can imagine yourself doing—something like skydiving or traveling to Tahiti. If your sex life has gotten into this rut, try using this chapter to help yourself break out of it.

Some of these suggestions may seem too romantic or "silly" to you at first, maybe all right for "young lovers" but not for you.

That's a mistake! Give romance a chance. You'll find that it can be fun and exciting once you get past your initial awkwardness. There is no rule that you have to give up romance and excitement at any age.

AN AFTERNOON DELIGHT

Instead of always making love at night, when one or both of you may be tired, try an "afternoon delight." You may be able to find time on the weekend, schedule some time off on a workday, take a long lunch hour, or use some other strategy. It may be more exciting if it's at a time when you wouldn't ordinarily be together.

Plan your afternoon dalliance at a time when you won't be disturbed. Unplug the phone. Perhaps this might be the time for lovemaking in or near the sunlight streaming through your window. Prepare your own little romantic island by spreading a quilt or furry rug on the floor in some interesting corner of your home and put on some music that you both enjoy.

To please your other senses for your afternoon adventure, arrange some fresh fruit, such as berries, grapes, orange slices, or cut melon, as well as your favorite cheese nearby. Select a light white wine or a sparkling water. Then, after some gentle caresses and a few sips of wine, enjoy your sensual adventure with whatever style of lovemaking you choose.

A FLORAL BOUQUET

Almost any woman, or man, will enjoy this enchanting experience. It can take place anytime or anyplace, although daylight is best, to fully benefit from the pleasurable visual effects.

The setting requires a bouquet of fresh flowers and a large, attractive bowl. Choose blooms with lots of soft petals and a variety of colors: daisies, carnations, roses, and others. Gently pull the petals off the flowers until the bowl is full of a medley of different hues.

Start off by sprinkling petals over your partner's closed eyes, face, body, and genital area. Make attractive designs, and let your partner's nipples poke through. Stroke his or her face and nipples with velvety rose petals, alternating with caresses. Gently slide the soft, silky petals around your partner's body, caressing through the satiny feel of the flowers.

If the two of you desire, you can switch places. Give your partner the pleasure of heaping the petals on you and caressing you through them. Then go ahead and make love in your bed full of flower petals. It will be an experience you won't forget.

A BUBBLE BATH FOR TWO

Playing in a sensuous bubble bath is a wonderful prelude to lovemaking. You may never have tried taking a bubble bath together, or you may have when you were younger but not in recent years.

A romantic atmosphere will help. Your bathroom will feel different if you use candlelight instead of the usual harsh, white bathroom light. You might like to have some wine or juice to sip. Grapes or orange slices are also good and can be handled with wet hands.

If there isn't enough room to sit facing each other, you can sit bobsled style, one behind the other. Enjoy the soothing, creamy feel of the bubbles and play with them while washing each other, caressing and touching. When you've had enough, towel each other dry gently. Use large, luxurious bath towels, if you have them. There is something very delicious about taking care of each other so nicely.

A bubble bath together can be enjoyed simply for its own sake, or it can serve as a relaxing introduction to lovemaking.

THE ROMANTIC BREAKFAST

You'll have to plan ahead for this gourmet feast, gathering some of the ingredients in advance. Use a weekend morning when you'll be at home, undisturbed, with plenty of time to spend. You won't want to be hurrying. Set the table for two, using your favorite place settings. This is an excellent time for your best china, silver, and linen napkins. A small bouquet of flowers or even just a single rose in a bud vase will add a loving touch.

Dress for breakfast as the two of you feel comfortable. On a warm summer day, some couples I've known like to dine in the nude or seminude. On the other hand, you might feel more comfortable in an attractive robe or have fun dressing up in formal clothes.

You might start your breakfast by sipping a delicious Mimosa Breeze, made with half orange juice and half champagne (or substitute a carbonated lemon-lime drink). Grenadine or maraschino cherry syrup can be added to taste. Garnish with a sprig of fresh mint, and serve with a cocktail straw.

Start a lighter menu with a fresh-fruit plate, and add a pastry and perhaps an egg dish. Another menu might include croissants and a caviar omelette capped with sour cream, a perfect romantic breakfast. Choose some soft music to complement the setting.

After the meal, it's back to bed to complete a leisurely morning. If you have privacy, open your blinds and let the sun shine in, or enjoy the sound of rain pattering on your windows. Proceed with lovemaking in whatever fashion seems right at the moment.

FEATHERING

Feathers are made for caressing. They are light, gentle, and soft, and feather caresses can be especially sensual and titillating. If possible, find three or four feathers of different sizes and consistencies. If not, a new, unused feather duster or two will do. Feathers have their own personalities: stiffer, pointed ones are best for tickling with the tip or edge, while softer, flowing ones are for gentle caresses.

With your partner on his or her back, start with soft, fluttery movements around the face and neck. Gradually move down to the chest and use flowing feather caresses to gently stroke the breasts and nipples. Men as well as women will enjoy this. Continue down your partner's thighs and abdomen. Stroking movements on the inner thigh can be very stimulating. Let your imagination run wild.

Using the feathers in this way can wonderfully tantalize your partner. You can find sensitive places on the back of the neck and in the cleavage of the backside, behind the knees and under the arms.

After a while, switch places so your partner can feather you. It's just as much fun to receive as to give, you'll find, and it will help you both to feel luxurious and pampered. It's a wonderful preparation for lovemaking.

LOVEMAKING WITH WARMED OIL

On cold winter nights few experiences are as sensuous as giving your partner a soft massage with warmed oil. This special treat tends to be most attractive when it's cold and wintery outside, but warm and toasty inside.

Prepare your room by creating a warm atmosphere. Candlelight's soft, flickering glow contributes to an overall sensual mood when you're giving a massage. A nice fire is a wonderful alternative. Add some soft music that you both enjoy. Some scented massage oils are made especially for oil rubs, but a kitchen oil such as corn oil or safflower oil will do as well.

Get ready by putting about a half cup of oil in a small bottle with a cap or stopper. A plastic bottle with a flip-top spout is best because you don't have to keep it upright; you can simply lay it down in your bed.

Warm the oil by placing the bottle in a sink full of hot water. Be sure to test the temperature of the oil before using it, though—and don't heat it on a stove or in a microwave, as oil can get too hot quickly.

When the oil is comfortably warm, it's time to begin. Either partner can go first and the exercise will be equally enjoyable, but let's describe the man doing the first caressing:

Have your partner lie on her stomach while you slide your fingers lightly up and down her back. Feel the texture of her skin, while she concentrates on the feel of your fingertips. Then pour a small amount of the warmed oil in the small of her back. Spread it out with your hand in ever-widening circles. Add more as you need to. Notice the changes in texture and sensation as oiled skin becomes smooth and silky. Your strokes and caresses will slide liquidly.

Try a variety of different touches. Use swirls, short strokes, and long strokes all up and down her back, and then light caresses with the tips of your fingers. Let your partner tell you what the caressing feels like and what feels best. Be slow and leisurely, take your time. Add a little more warm oil from time to time to keep the warmth and the silky feeling.

Now pour a small amount of oil on her buttocks and the backs of her thighs, and let your hands teasingly play with these more sexually sensitive areas. Then spread her legs a little, cup a little of the warm oil in your hand, and, after making sure that it's not too warm, apply it gently to her vulva.

Lubricating her vaginal area with the warm oil will add to her arousal as well as yours. The inside of her vaginal lips and her vaginal opening will be soft and warm, silky and wet. You can make small, circular movements with one or two fingers inside her vaginal lips and around her clitoris while your other hand continues to slide up and down her back. This can provide her with a most enjoyable combination—enjoying a back rub and having her genital area stimulated at the same time. Then reach between her legs and slide your hand through her wet vulval area. It will feel delightfully velvety with the oil.

Switch hands or take a break by caressing her back and sides again. Then put some more oil in your hand and return to her genital area.

To her: You may already be quite aroused, but if the two of you can wait, you may wish to caress your partner with the oil in the same way. You can begin by giving him a back massage, stroking his buttocks and between his legs. Or just start by having him turn over on his back while you help him get hard by putting some of the warm oil in your hand and caressing his penis and scrotum. You'll enjoy sliding your hands up and down his slippery penis, and he'll think it's great. It will give him a double sensation if you cup his scrotum in one hand while you stroke his penis with the other.

Once you are both aroused and your partner is hard, you'll enjoy straddling him and sliding his penis into your vagina. After playing in this position for a while, roll over; with your bodies slippery with oil, intercourse in a face-to-face position will have an added dimension as your entire bodies slide against each other. You will especially enjoy the feeling of your partner's chest sliding against your breasts as his penis thrusts in and out of your vagina.

Making love with warm oil is an experience you can enjoy and come back to over and over again. It will be a delightful addition to your lovemaking choices.

LOVEMAKING WITH MIRRORS

Making love in front of a mirror can add to your feelings of intimacy and arousal while you share the stimulation of seeing your own sexual responses.

If you'd like to try this interesting variation, we suggest you prepare a suitable atmosphere in advance. A couple of candles set at the far ends of a mirror and reflecting in it can create a beautiful setting. And as always, some soft music will complement the mood.

A mirror across the room is probably too far away. If you're ten feet from the mirror, your image seems twenty feet away. If you have to strain to see yourself, you've lost the effect.

More than likely, your house won't have a movable mirror, so consider spreading a quilt on the floor in front of a fixed mirror to experiment. If this isn't convenient, try making love in front of one of the large mirrors found over bathroom counters or dressing tables. You might want to place a pillow or two on the countertop to lean on for comfort.

Begin by standing together in the nude in front of the mirror. Caress your partner and cup her breasts in your hands while you both enjoy the view of your bodies with the candlelight flickering on you. Lubricate her vaginal area with a little warm lovemaking oil. Your partner can help you to get hard by playing with your penis and applying some lubricant to it—and she may enjoy licking your penis or sucking on it while you both watch. Seeing your bodies in the candlelight and watching the preparation can build a delicious sexual tension for both of you.

Let your partner lean forward over the counter or dressing table and rest her arms and head on a pillow for comfort. As you stand behind her, caress her buttocks and labia and then spread her vaginal lips and run your fingers softly around her vaginal opening and over her clitoris. Slide your penis inside her and place your hand on her hips to guide your movements while you both enjoy watching your bodies move in rhythm to the music. You'll be surprised at how arousing this can be.

If the two of you shift around slightly to stand at an angle to the mirror, you'll get a good view of each other and your body movements, which will look especially attractive in the flickering candlelight. Standing sideways to the mirror like this will give your partner a better view. She may even be able to see your penis sliding in and out of her vagina. If by any chance you have a second mirror that you can set at an angle (on the bathroom door, for instance), you'll be able to observe your lovemaking from several different directions.

Many people find it extraordinarily stimulating to watch themselves in a mirror and see the beauty of their bodies in action. Others feel that it's not as pleasurable as the "close in bed" atmosphere that they are accustomed to in lovemaking. If you've never tried it, I suggest you do so at least once—if only to discover that you really look surprisingly attractive during sex.

THE EXTENDED BREAST CARESS

Caressing your partner's breasts can be a prelude to intercourse, or it can be a lovemaking art form all its own. It can vary from a little "good morning" lick of her nipple to an extended erotic caress. It can be very sexually exciting, or else soothing and relaxing, depending on the mood and circumstances.

To begin, choose a time when you are at leisure and unhurried. Gradually start making love to one of your partner's breasts as you lie alongside her. I say "making love" to one of her breasts, because that's what you'll do. You'll give that breast the most wonderfully complete, loving attention it's ever had.

Start by gently licking around the base of her breast, and with gradual swirls of your tongue work your way toward her nipple. Tease a little by playing near her nipple with your tongue, retreating and returning to it. As your partner's nipples become erect and seem to reach out for your caress, try the lightest of touches— with a cotton ball, Q-Tip, feather, or filmy, smooth material. Blow on her nipple and touch it ever so lightly with the tip of your tongue.

Watch the nipple react as you flick it with your tongue, suck on it gently, or bathe it softly with your open lips or the fullness of your soft tongue. Dip a little wine or your favorite after-dinner liqueur on the nipple with a cotton ball or your finger and lick it off.

Cup her breast with both of your hands and bring her nipple up to your mouth as you continue to bathe it with your tongue. Try different kinds of strokes, licking softly over the nipple, taking it entirely in your mouth and rolling it with your tongue, or making swirling movements around it. Run the erect nipple between your lips or gently between your fingers. Cup one hand over it and let it tickle your palm.

You may find that you're giving attention to your partner's breast for twenty to thirty minutes. It can be a really ecstatic experience for her, especially if she knows that you're enjoying it too. In fact, you may get an earnest request to do the same on the other side, thereby doubling the fun for both of you.

This breast stimulation can be an end in itself. You can give your partner a nipple bath with your tongue before dropping off to sleep, or you can waken her in the morning with some nipple licks, just for fun.

On the other hand, you can continue stimulating her breasts with your tongue and lips while one of your fingers slips into her vulval opening. You can then give your partner double stimulation, caressing her clitoris and nipple at the same time, until you finish by having intercourse, a wonderful conclusion to this delightful adventure.

A LITTLE INSURANCE

When you have one of these romantic adventures planned, with a lot of preparation and anticipation, you may feel some unexpected pressure to perform, especially if you and your partner have been looking forward to the lovemaking and talking about how much fun it will be. If you have any worry about disappointing your partner, discussing it in advance will help. This would also be an ideal time to use a small dose of Viagra as insurance to allow you to be confident that you will get erect with no difficulty. (See chapter 2, "The Viagra Revolution.") That way you can plan one of these little adventures without any nagging worry about embarrassment in the back of your mind.

AND A FINAL HINT

Do you find yourself thinking about lovemaking when you get up, feeling sexual tingling in the morning, joking with your friends or business associates about sex during the day, looking forward to it at dinner—but then all too often feeling, as you get in bed late at night, that your body is tired and ready for sleep and desire has disappeared?

As the years have gone by, you've probably noticed that you simply tire out earlier in the evening, while lovemaking continues to require energy, creativity, and enthusiasm. If late at night, after the evening news, is when you usually plan your sex life, just plain weariness can often cause disappointment and take most of the enjoyment out of it. By evening you're likely to be preoccupied with the concerns, annoyances, and anxieties of the day, and this stress, as well as simple fatigue, makes the transition to a sexual mood a difficult one.

Lovemaking in the morning gives you the opportunity to make love when your body is rested and your mind is fresh and clear. It has real advantages for men and women over forty, and it can make sex a pleasure instead of a chore.

There will be some days when you simply don't have the opportunity to lie in bed for any length of time. On other occasions, however, you may be able to arrange for leisurely awakening and the luxury of morning lovemaking. You can proceed imperceptibly from closeness and touching during sleep to gradual cuddling, hugging, and caressing. As your lovemaking begins, you may feel extremely sensual, close, and intimate, as if in the continuation of a pleasant dream.

Even on mornings when you have to arise fairly early, you can still enjoy a sensuous "appetizer" together. A few minutes of intimate love play can help establish a feeling of excitement and closeness that lasts throughout the day. There is no need for either of you to climax. It can just be a quick reminder of your love and affection for each other.

CHAPTER 8

UNDERSTANDING YOUR
OLDER MAN

If you are a woman whose partner is experiencing some of the sexual changes of aging, there are a lot of things that you can do to help him, as well as yourself, enjoy sex more fully. By assisting him in achieving and maintaining firmer erections during lovemaking, you will also be reassuring him of how much you care for him at a time when he may be experiencing great insecurity about his attractiveness and masculinity as well as his sexual performance.

Anxiety about performance can turn a man's natural changes of aging into real sexual dysfunction. If your partner's sexual changes are compounded by medical conditions that interfere with his erection, you may not be able to entirely overcome these problems yourself. You will, however, certainly be able to alleviate whatever part of his problem is caused by worry over his sexual performance and his need for loving sexual stimulation.

Now that your partner is forty, fifty, or older, he no longer has the same sexual response as he did when he was twenty. As a very young man, his sexual drive was so strong that he could usually perform under the least conducive of conditions. He could get erect in awkward, cramped positions in the backseat of a car. He could still get erect after a half dozen beers. He would even manage to get erect when you didn't want sex and weren't responsive at all.

If you think back on those years when your partner got hard just seeing you in the nude or thinking about the two of you making love, it's tempting to blame yourself and wonder, "Has he lost interest in me?" "Is he bored with me?" or even "Is he having an affair with someone else?"

Of course, any of these developments may be true, but the fact that he's no longer springing to erection just seeing you undressed doesn't necessarily imply those things at all. He may very well still find you attractive and care deeply about you. However, his lack of spontaneous erections is simply a natural result of aging. And just as your partner's eyes may now need some help from eyeglasses, his penis needs some help with *direct physical stmulation* from you.

It may be just as simple as that: Not a loss of interest in you. Not that he's having an affair. Not necessarily a need for Viagra. Just that he needs your physical help to get hard.

HE MAY SEEM TO HAVE LOST
INTEREST IN SEX

A common complaint I've encountered in my practice treating sexual dysfunctions is "He doesn't seem interested in sex anymore." Women often report that they and their partners are having sexual relations quite infrequently: once in two weeks, once a month, even less than that. These women want to have sex more frequently, but they say they can't get their partners interested.

In these circumstances it often turns out that the woman's partner hasn't really lost interest in sex at all. The real problem is that he's become insecure about his erection ability and worried about his sexual performance. He's afraid to initiate sex because he's worried that he won't be able to get hard if he does, and he's afraid of the embarrassment if he can't.

HOW PERFORMANCE ANXIETY CAN AFFECT HIS SEX LIFE

It's astounding the amount of apprehension and worry your partner may develop if he's had a few repeated episodes of difficulty. Erection problems are often worsened by this performance anxiety, and the two may work together to create a vicious circle. Your partner may start feeling apprehension before the lovemaking even starts. The more anxiety he has, and the more he mentally watches himself to see if he's getting hard, the more trouble he'll actually have and the more difficult it will be for him not to worry the next time.

WOMEN HAVE A BIG ADVANTAGE IN LOVEMAKING

Women are used to fluctuation in their own level of excitement. They know that they may become very aroused during lovemaking on some occasions and not quite as excited on others, and that excitement levels may vary during the lovemaking sessions themselves. Women generally tend to take this fluctuation for granted and don't react with much concern if they are less responsive at one time than another. For this reason, it may be hard for you, as a woman, to understand why your male partner gets so upset when he's less responsive and has difficulty getting an erection.

You have a big advantage being a woman. You can begin love-making and proceed to intercourse even if you're preoccupied, worried, or not very excited. You can start even if you're not lubricated. It may not be very satisfactory to you, but you can do it if you want to: if, for instance, you want to please your partner, even though you aren't feeling sexy yourself. You may, of course, then become more excited once you've begun.

On the other hand, if your partner is worried or preoccupied, he probably won't be able to get an erection to begin with. And if he can't get erect, he is simply unable to go ahead with intercourse.

Try to imagine how he feels: He wants very much to get an erection and feels that you'll be disappointed if he doesn't. He probably feels that an erection is necessary for lovemaking (although it's not), yet he himself has no control over it. He can't *make* himself get hard any more than you can *make* yourself get wet vaginally.

In fact, vaginal lubrication for a woman is in many ways the equivalent of getting erect for a man. It is a natural response to sexual stimulation, when it's not blocked by anxiety or other negative emotions. Imagine if you *had* to get wet in order to have intercourse! There isn't any way to *make* yourself lubricate, of course. The harder you "tried," the more trouble you'd be likely to have. And if you couldn't get wet on one occasion, you would probably worry even more the next time.

If that sounds nightmarish to you, realize that older men often feel that they are under that kind of pressure to perform. The stress is sometimes so bad that they just give up on sex completely rather than endure any more embarrassment or feelings of failure.

IT'S NOT BECAUSE HE DOESN'T
FIND YOU ATTRACTIVE

As we mentioned before, your partner's difficulty in becoming aroused most probably has nothing to do with any lack of sexual interest in you, but instead reflects that his body is now simply less spontaneous in translating sexual interest into an erection. His penis now requires stroking in order to get hard.

Realizing and accepting this will enable you to put aside any feelings of resentment or insecurity and allow you to be the caring, helping, and loving sexual partner that you would like to be. Remember, you have a choice: You can ignore his needs and possibly create a wall or barrier between the two of you, or you can assist him and greatly add to the intimacy, warmth, and love of your relationship.

COOPERATION AND
UNDERSTANDING ARE CRUCIAL

Often in my practice I see two older men with the same potential sexual ability. One of them is functioning well and enjoying a satisfying and successful sex life. The other thinks that he's impotent, or partly impotent, and is frustrated and unhappy. The primary difference between them may be that the first man has a cooperative, understanding partner who cheerfully helps him to function, while the second man's partner is uncooperative and negative about sex. This is no exaggeration; a man's partner can easily make that much difference.

Your attitude will be very important to your mutual success in maintaining a healthy sex life. It's important to curb irritation or resentment if your partner has sexual difficulties. Demanding that your partner get an erection in order to make love will only put additional performance pressure on him, which will make him even less likely to function in the way that you desire. It simply won't get you what you want, and will actually be counterproductive.

ALLOW YOUR PARTNER TO BE A GOOD LOVER EVEN WITHOUT AN ERECTION

If your partner has trouble on a particular occasion, it will work much better if you cheerfully accept having him pleasure you manually or orally. This will achieve a much better result than insisting on intercourse as your exclusive means of sexual gratification. It will give your partner the feeling that he can satisfy you and be a good lover whether or not his penis gets hard. This will decrease his anxiety and his pressure for performance, and it will probably make it easier for him to get hard without worry the next time you make love.

Many a man whom I've seen in my practice with erection problems has told me that his partner won't allow him to bring her to climax by manual or oral means if he can't get hard. Sometimes it's because she thinks he doesn't really want to. Other women feel, misguidedly, that "it's not natural" or confuse sexual stimulation by their partner with masturbation, which of course usually refers to self-stimulation.

It's really a mistake to turn down your partner's attempts to please you manually. In doing so, you're giving him a message that the only way he can really please you is by getting hard, and that message puts a great deal of pressure on him.

Now that your partner's erection mechanism is more fragile, your cooperation and help will be very important. And there is nothing that will make an older man more appreciative than having a partner who helps to restore his erection ability. I'll explore more about specific practical ways you can help your partner in the next chapter.

CHAPTER 9

HOW TO HELP YOUR MAN GET FIRM ERECTIONS

PREPARING

If your partner is like many older men, he will usually be able to get erect when conditions are favorable, but he may have difficulty when they're not. Therefore, it can help if the two of you try to establish a sensuous, nondistracting environment for lovemaking. You can do this by dimming the lights, adding soft music, and disconnecting the telephone, for example.

It's a mistake to make love only late at night, when you're both fatigued. Your partner will probably get erect more easily when you are both rested in the morning. Mid-afternoon on a relaxed weekend is another good time. Lovemaking when your partner is under high stress or when both of you are feeling pressured may result in temporary erection difficulties. It may take a little while for your partner to get erect under the best of circumstances. Allow adequate time whenever possible so that neither of you feels rushed.

It's a good idea to have a lubricant on hand. Extra lubrication can be a valuable aid for penetration when your partner's erection isn't as fully hard as you both might wish. (A lubricant made for lovemaking such as Astroglide is best, but in an emergency a simple kitchen oil such as corn oil will do.)

STARTING LOVEMAKING

It's important that you both realize that it isn't necessary for your partner to have an erection before starting lovemaking. The erection will come later with mutual stimulation.

Many couples begin lovemaking with simultaneous hugging, caressing, and petting. However, it's often helpful to *take turns* caressing each other. Your partner may sometimes want to bring you to a climax with manual or oral petting even before you start caressing him. Helping you climax may reassure him that he can satisfy you with or without an erection, and may thus allow him to be less anxious about getting hard. Men often worry a great deal about their sexual function, and worrying about getting hard enough to satisfy you can certainly interfere with his getting erect.

When you start to caress him, let him know that it's his turn to relax and enjoy. Remind him that he doesn't need to worry about getting hard because you really enjoy making love with him and he can give you lots of sexual pleasure, whether or not he gets an erection on this particular occasion.

Assuming that your lover has recently had difficulty with erections, you can begin your arousal of him by having him lie on his stomach and giving him a gentle overall body massage to help him relax. This is also a very nondemanding position for him.

The massage can be accompanied by stroking over his buttocks and sliding your hand gently between his legs to stroke the back of his scrotum and the base of his penis from behind.

When your partner rolls over on his back, continue with light stroking movements between his thighs and along his scrotum and penis. Use very light touches on his scrotum, because the testicles are very sensitive.

The most sexually sensitive places for a man are usually the underside of his penis and the ridge below the head of his penis (the coronal ridge). The little indentation of that ridge on the underside of the penis is called the frenulum and is extra-sensitive. If the man is uncircumcised, the foreskin will retract as he becomes erect and the head of his penis, which will be exposed, will be especially sensitive.

CARING AND TENDER CARESSES

Approach caressing with an artistic and creative attitude. You'll want to do the best, most sensuous, most imaginative job you can. Being caring and tender, however, is most important of all. Softly stroke and caress your partner's inner thighs, slip the tips of your fingers lightly along the hairs of his scrotum, and slide your fingertips or your tongue down the underside of the shaft of his penis. Softly cup his scrotum in your hand as you stroke his penis with your other hand.

Now begin sliding your hand up and down the whole shaft of your partner's penis, swirling or slipping over and around the coronal ridge. A gentle rhythmic pulling movement on the shaft and head of his penis will also help him to get hard. You can do this either with your hand or with your mouth.

Use your imagination to picture what your partner would enjoy, and ask him to give you feedback and let you know what excites him. Remember, too, that just as you may vary from day to day in the touches that feel just right to you, the same may be true for him.

STIMULATE HIS PENIS USING
A SEXUAL LUBRICANT

Using a sexual lubricant on your partner's penis will feel very sensuous to him, as if you were applying suntan oil or baby oil. Sometimes it may feel cold if applied directly from the bottle, so you might warm it in your hands first. Or place the container in some hot water in your sink. The oil will help your hands slide up and down without irritating his penis. The wet, warm, slippery sensation will create a feeling similar to the one he gets when his penis is inside your vagina.

A sexual lubricant can really make a *BIG* difference in helping a man with erection difficulties to respond. Don't ignore this suggestion.

Be gentle but firm when playing with your partner's penis. After you have applied a lubricant, you can try different kinds of stimulation, such as sliding the penis between the palms of your hands laid flat, as if you were rolling a stick or a piece of dough. You can use one hand to hold the base of the shaft while you slide the other up and down over the coronal ridge. You might try using just the tips of your fingers. Remember to ask your partner what kinds of touches he likes best.

Many men find that long strokes up and down the shaft of the penis are important in helping it to get hard, while touches around the exquisitely sensitive ridge (equivalent, perhaps, to your clitoris) help bring him to climax. There is a tremendous overlap, however, between the two kinds of sensations, either of which may work best at different times.

Most older men also find that oral stimulation of the penis is especially valuable in helping them get hard. I'll discuss this more in the next chapter.

HIS NIPPLES MAY BE ESPECIALLY SENSITIVE

Two important areas of a man's body that are often overlooked are his nipples. You can lick your partner's nipples or touch them with your fingertips while you're simultaneously stroking his penis. They can be quite sensitive—even as sensitive as yours. Your partner may tell you that the sensation goes right from his nipple to the tip of his penis, if you are stroking his penis at the same time.

Nipple stimulation can be especially important *as an aid to ejaculation.* If, on some occasions, he finds that he just can't climax during intercourse or even during manual stimulation, lightly flicking or pinching his nipples at the same time may provide the necessary extra stimulation that he needs.

WHAT IF HE CONTINUES TO BE ANXIOUS?

Don't get discouraged if your partner doesn't get erect in the first minute or two. He may be dealing with a lot of anxiety and also may be wondering how you feel about caressing him. Before he can relax enough to let an erection happen, he needs to feel secure and confident in you, to realize that you enjoy making love to him, and to know that you won't be angry or annoyed if he fails to get erect.

If he continues to worry or seems preoccupied with anxiety, try to distract him with sexual thoughts. Get him to talk to you and tell you what your hands and mouth feel like on his penis, or have him recall a specifically exciting lovemaking episode the two of you enjoyed together. Tell him to describe it to you in detail. This will help him focus his attention sexually.

As an alternative, you might talk to him while you stroke him. Tell him what his penis feels like, how good it feels to you, or what its texture is like when you stroke it or lick it and feel it growing. Another choice would be to tell him your favorite sex fantasy or reminisce about a particularly exciting lovemaking session and what it felt like for you. If he concentrates on what you're saying, it will certainly take his mind off worrying, and this will allow your sexual stimulation to do its job and make him hard.

When you find a method of stimulation that works, remember it for the next time he has difficulty. Using a method that he knows has worked before will give him more confidence, both in your ability to help him and in his own ability to get hard.

WHAT IF HIS ERECTION GOES DOWN?

In most cases, the kinds of caressing that we have described above will enable your partner to have a good erection, provided he doesn't have a medical problem. Now that your partner is over forty, however, it may take him some time before he can climax, and his erection itself may not last that long. In fact, his erection may go down at perplexing and sometimes inexplicable times—such as right in the middle of intercourse.

When your partner loses his erection, he may tend to get discouraged and disgusted with himself and feel humiliated. He may also believe that he can't get hard again once his first erection is gone. Therefore, if your partner has been having trouble with maintaining his erection, he may hurry to try to use it as soon as he gets hard. This will add to his anxiety and may cause him to lose his erection even more quickly.

There is really no need for the momentary loss of erection to be a problem. It depends entirely on how the two of you deal with it. There is no earthly reason why one erection has to last for the whole time of lovemaking. If your partner loses his first erection, he can have a second or third later in that lovemaking episode, especially if you help him regain it.

USE THE TEASING TECHNIQUE TO BUILD HIS CONFIDENCE

An easy technique, one that is frequently used in sexual therapy, can help you build your partner's confidence and assist him in dealing with occasional loss of erection. It's called the *Teasing Technique*, and here's how it works:

Start by agreeing beforehand that you won't have intercourse during this exercise—even if your partner gets the world's hardest erection. This will ease performance pressure. He won't have to worry that he's not going to get hard enough to penetrate, since you won't be going on to intercourse anyway. When he does start to get hard, he won't be preoccupied, worrying that he may lose his erection before he can complete the lovemaking.

Let your partner lie back and relax. Gradually run your fingertips around his penis. Then lick and pull it with your lips, as I described earlier in the chapter, or lubricate it with your favorite sexual lubricant and gently stroke it with your hands until your partner gets erect.

When he does, keep playing with his penis but don't bring him to a climax and don't go on to intercourse. Then, after a little while, just stop and let his erection go back down! This may seem like a strange thing to do, but you're going to help him get and lose his erection several times today.

In the past, when he was worried about keeping his erection, he may have lost it easily. Now, when you want it to go down, it may be obstinate and refuse. In this case, it's okay to play a little and act silly—tickle him, sprinkle water on his penis, make him laugh. Then, when his erection has finally gone down, you can return and get him aroused again or else take a break and let him caress you.

After a brief rest, help him to get hard again, and then let his erection go down again. Repeat this process a few times, with short breaks in between. You will both be amazed at how many times he can get erect, as long as he hasn't reached a climax.

When you are ready to conclude your lovemaking, decide whether or not you will bring him to a climax with oral or manual stimulation. He may be happy just with the repeated excitation and wish to save his climax for a subsequent lovemaking experience later that day or the next, when the two of you may wish to have full intercourse. Your own climax can come either before or after his.

The series of erections that you help your partner get and then lose in one lovemaking episode will help him realize that losing his erection isn't the end of the world. He'll know that he has the capacity for many erections, and that at his age having erections come and go is just a natural part of the lovemaking process, not any kind of crisis.

Repeat the Teasing Technique at least once a week for three or four weeks to build his confidence. Do this exercise in addition to your regular lovemaking. After a while, if your partner loses his erection during intercourse, he'll know that you will help him to get it back, most of the time, lovingly and without complaint. This reassurance will help him to function as well as he possibly can. There will inevitably be an occasional time when his erection won't come back, no matter what. Don't try to force it. There's always another time!

IN SUMMARY

It's my impression that *at least* 80 to 85 percent of older men with erection problems have some underlying physical problem contributing to making their erections more fragile, primarily the result of arteriosclerosis. Often, though, there is a combination of physical and emotional factors, with the physical problems causing initial difficulty and anxiety worsening the problem.

Most older men will respond very well to the simple, helpful methods described in these last two chapters. If, however, in spite of your best efforts, your partner's erection problems persist, there are two possible explanations.

The first is that he may have a medical problem due to illness, medication side effects, lack of hormones, more severe vascular difficulties, or other physical problems that I will examine in subsequent chapters. In this case, he will need a medical evaluation.

The other possibility is that his erection fragility is causing a great deal of anxiety about his sexual functioning that has not yet been eliminated by your reassurance and caressing. This becomes a vicious circle as the more he worries the more fragile the erection will be, and it is very difficult for him to break this circle himself.

If the problem is primarily due to anxiety, taking Viagra on a few occasions will overcome the anxiety and produce erections in spite of any worry he may be feeling. This will break the cycle of anxiety and reassure your partner that his problem won't mean he'll be impotent forever, which is probably what he is fearing. After he has functioned well with the Viagra on several occasions, he will probably do fine without it, just knowing that he has it in reserve in case of problems.

If the problem is due to other medical problems, it is also almost certain that some treatment will be available that can restore his ability to function. Viagra is only one of many alternatives. We explore them in chapter 25, "How We Treat Erection Problems."

CHAPTER 10

HOW AN OLDER WOMAN
CAN HELP HER PARTNER'S
ERECTIONS BY USING
ORAL SEX

Although I have mentioned oral lovemaking several times in previous chapters, I am all too aware that many older women are still uncomfortable with it. However it is such an effective method for encouraging good erections and maintaining mutual enjoyment that I am devoting this entire chapter to exploring it. You may very well find that greater knowledge will allow you to have increased confidence, less inhibition, and, ultimately, success and pleasure in this important technique.

Even if you think you will never be able to use oral lovemaking because of long conditioning against it, try reading the chapter anyway. Reading it doesn't commit you to anything, and, who knows, you may decide to experiment.

HE MAY NEED THE EXTRA STIMULATION

As I've stressed before, an older man needs more direct stimulation in order to achieve good erections. Oral stimulation is a very effective way to help. It's also a tender and intimate way to show your feelings of caring.

In my treatment of sexual dysfunction, couples often came to me because the man was no longer getting spontaneous erections. This difficulty usually occured sometime in the man's forties or fifties, when he started needing more direct stimulation to get hard. Embarrassed by his lack of spontaneous erections, he may have even started avoiding sex. His partner was often unhappy about the lack of physical contact, but in spite of this she may still have rejected the idea of using mouth caresses to help.

They both missed out by this refusal. She missed a chance to help her partner and to show her love and affection in a tender and pleasurable way. He failed to get a delightful form of stimulation that might have assisted him to have better and more frequent erections. And they both lost the chance to continue to enjoy lovemaking and have intercourse in a happy and mutually rewarding way.

IT MAY BE DIFFICULT TO TALK ABOUT

Young couples now take oral petting for granted as a natural part of their lovemaking. Recent studies of sexual practices show that oral sex is as common as sexual intercourse in the lovemaking of young adults. On the other hand, many men and women over fifty or sixty have lots of inhibitions and taboos about it.

If you've never used *fellatio* (stimulating your partner's penis with your mouth), you may wonder what your partner would think if you tried it. Many older couples find that it's difficult to talk about. The man hesitates to ask for it because he's afraid his partner might be offended. The woman fears that if she initiates it her partner will be shocked. So neither of them brings it up.

And so, many women in their fifties, sixties, or older who have tried fellatio have used it hesitantly and unsurely. Caroline R., a fifty-five-year-old woman, told me that she really wanted to help her husband but didn't know how to use oral sex. "I'm not sure what Bill would like, or how much pressure to use. I'm afraid of hurting him with my teeth or just doing it wrong. I want both of us to enjoy it, but I guess I just don't know how to begin."

Depending on your age, and your parents' attitudes when you were growing up, you may have been raised with many inhibitions about your own genitals, to say nothing of a man's. You may have been raised with the idea that your genital area was dirty and shouldn't even be touched. This kind of indoctrination can make you feel very squeamish about oral lovemaking.

SKIN IS SKIN AND CLEAN IS CLEAN!

With regard to the issue of cleanliness of the penis and the scrotum, it's important to realize that skin is just skin. The skin on your partner's penis is no different from the skin on his arm or elbow. If it's clean, it's clean.

Actually, your mouth has immeasurably more bacteria than the skin on a freshly washed penis. If you're worried about sterility, it would make more sense to give up kissing than fellatio.

You've probably heard a lot of vulgar names for oral sex, but you've probably heard an even greater number of vulgar names for sexual intercourse. So don't let the vocabulary put you off from oral lovemaking unless you're prepared to give up intercourse, too.

IT CAN BE FUN FOR YOU, TOO

Although you may be apprehensive about oral lovemaking, it may help you to know that many, if not most, women find it very enjoyable and erotic for themselves, and not just for their partner.

Your mouth, after all, is a very erogenous organ. That's why you enjoy kissing so much. You can get the same feelings of excitement from fellatio.

Think of your partner's penis as your own private plaything. Enjoy its texture and feel, as well as your ability to make it grow. Think of it as a sign of your power that with your tongue and lips you can make this soft, small penis grow to be big, full, and firm. You'll find that you will come to enjoy the feel of the penis in your mouth, just as your partner enjoys the feel of your nipple and breast in his.

HOW SHOULD I BEGIN?

If using your mouth to stimulate your partner's penis is relatively new to you, you may wonder how to begin. Let me suggest a plan drawn from some of my patients' experiences.

You can reassure yourself about cleanliness beforehand by showering together and washing your partner's penis with soap and water. Remember: When it's washed, it's clean. Showering together has another advantage, as it can also be a romantic start to lovemaking.

Then begin by having your partner lie on his back and gently kiss him along his stomach and legs while you caress his penis

with your hands. Then brush your lips along the shaft of his pe-·
nis with very light kisses at first. This will help you to get accustomed to the feel of it and sort of reassure you that it won't bite.

Now, slowly and gently slide your tongue up and down the underside of the shaft of his penis. As you feel more confident, you
can use your tongue to make short licks across the shaft as well as
up and down it. The underside of the shaft and the ridge around
the head of the penis are especially sensitive.

Using a flavored treat (such as a small amount of chocolate
syrup) on your partner's penis can be a help in getting over any
initial reluctance to oral lovemaking. It may be a little sticky, but
if you enjoy the taste enough you won't mind the stickiness at all.

Intersperse licks with gentle kisses. Play your tongue around
the ridge near the tip. Flick the little indentation where the ridge
meets the underside of the shaft with your tongue. Let the tip of
the penis slide into your mouth, and swirl your tongue around it.
This will feel very warm, wet, and sensual to your partner, like
having his penis caressed with hot, wet velvet.

Many women who are reluctant at first are amazed to discover
how much they enjoy this kind of lovemaking *themselves*. Sixty-
year-old Elizabeth W., who had been married for thirty-five years,
told me, "I used to think oral sex was something I could never do.
I only tried it to help Herb. I felt he really needed me. Now I'm
surprised to find out how good it feels to me to play with his penis in my mouth. I never would have believed it."

YOU'LL ENJOY BEING CREATIVE
AND PLAYFUL

It's not necessary to try to take the *entire* penis into your mouth.
It's much more important to be creative, loving, enthusiastic, and

playful. It's fun to be in control of giving your partner such pleasure.

Gradually add slight sucking movements by pulling with your
lips as you slide up on the penis. As Elizabeth W. found out, this
can be stimulating for you, too. Your lips and tongue are two of
your most important sensual organs.

Delight in the various sensations of your lips and mouth in
contact with your partner's penis and scrotum. The skin of his penis will feel very soft and wrinkly at first. You'll notice the texture
changing as you cause his erection to harden. His skin will feel
smoother and more velvety to your lips as his penis grows in size.
Notice which areas feel best to your lips and which are more exciting to your tongue.

USE YOUR MOUTH AND HAND
TOGETHER FOR ADDED PLEASURE

Your partner will be very conscious of the warmth and wetness of
your lips and tongue on his penis. If you gently fondle his scrotum at the same time with your hand, it will add a new focus of
pleasure.

You can give him even more sensations by initially using your
mouth alone, and then adding stimulation with your hand by sliding it up and down the shaft of his penis while your mouth is
pulling gently or swirling around its head.

Your partner will find the oral stimulation and the wetness of
your lips and tongue to be very exciting. But if you use your lips
too lightly he may not get enough sensation. Without the additional stimulation of your hand sliding up and down the shaft of
his penis, he may have trouble getting fully hard or climaxing.

It's normal for your jaws to get tired after a while, especially as it's necessary to keep your mouth fairly wide open to keep your teeth out of the way. Scraping the penis with your teeth can be very distracting, and your partner may well lose his erection. Cushion your teeth by slightly curling your lips over them. If your jaw does get tired, just pause and stimulate your partner with your hand for a while before resuming your oral caresses.

"AM I DOING IT RIGHT?"

What's "right"? Women often wonder if they are performing oral sex "correctly." There isn't any such thing as *correctly*. It's a question of what feels good to your partner, and the best way to find out is to ask him. And don't feel hurt if he asks you to do it a little bit differently than you have been. How can you know what feels best *to him* unless he tells you.

HAVING YOUR PARTNER CLIMAX DURING ORAL SEX IS OPTIONAL

Many men find that climaxing during oral stimulation is very intense and pleasurable. Some women, in turn, delight in having their partner climax while in their mouths, while others don't enjoy this sensation or else enjoy it only occasionally. Those who enjoy it find feeling the contractions of their partner's penis and continuing to stimulate it with their mouth during his climax to be intensely arousing. Others enjoy giving their partner pleasure with oral petting but may not want him to climax while they're doing it. It's solely a matter of individual preference.

You can be assured that your partner will have enough warning to let you know when he is about to climax, in case you don't want him to do so while his penis is in your mouth. You will feel the contractions of his penis a second or two before he ejaculates as well. If you want to withdraw your mouth at that time, make sure to continue stimulation by sliding your hand up and down his penis. It would be very disconcerting to your partner to have all stimulation stop abruptly, just as his climax is starting.

Semen is a simple liquid containing a number of substances you consume and digest every day: protein, calcium, citric acid, and cholesterol, among others. It usually has very little taste. Some women find the taste of semen pleasant and arousing. Others prefer to follow it with a sweet or pungent substance such as wine or fruit. Certain foods, such as garlic, can impart their taste to a man's semen.

ORAL LOVEMAKING IS LESS PHYSICALLY STRESSFUL

An advantage of fellatio is that it requires much less physical exertion than intercourse does. It can be used in most cases, even if one of you is particularly fatigued or not feeling completely well. This can be especially important if stress to the heart is a concern. It can also be a useful way of making love to your partner if illness, arthritis, or some other problem makes you temporarily unable to enjoy intercourse yourself.

YOUR PARTNER CAN START BY STIMULATING YOU

A nice alternative is to have your male partner begin the lovemaking session by orally stimulating you (see chapter 11). He can continue until you climax, or else he can stop at an earlier stage, whatever the two of you desire.

You can then use oral caresses to help him to get hard, and from there go on to intercourse. If you don't climax during intercourse but remain stimulated afterward, your partner can bring you to climax at that point.

While it's nice on occasion to have mutual oral lovemaking, it's certainly not necessary or even desirable every time. You and your partner should feel flexible about it, so that, depending on the circumstances of your lovemaking encounter, your partner may orally stimulate you, you may orally stimulate him, or you may both use oral caresses on each other.

Many couples enjoy experimenting with simultaneous oral lovemaking, which is sometimes referred to as "sixty-nine." You can do this with either of you kneeling over the other, with each having his or her head toward the other's genitals. Many people enjoy making love this way, but others find that it can be distracting. It may become difficult to concentrate on what you're doing when you are receiving such intense stimulation.

So oral stimulation can be as varied as intercourse. It can be engaged in just for fun, as a prelude to intercourse, to help your partner get hard, or to bring him to a climax. Use it as an added ingredient in your lovemaking, to be experienced and enjoyed in different ways at different times.

ORAL LOVEMAKING: AS OLD AS THE HILLS

Oral sex is not some new kinky idea that has just been dreamed up. Oral-genital contact has been a part of sexuality throughout history. Paintings and sculptures from ancient China, Japan, Greece, South America, and Africa show how universal this practice has always been. Yet today we continue to harbor many taboos and inhibitions about it. It's even theoretically illegal in some places.

Actually, using your mouth to give pleasure to your partner is one of the most gentle and intimate ways of expressing sexual love and showing your affection. Values have changed and are continuing to do so to reflect the universality of oral lovemaking. Marriage and sex manuals now devote whole chapters to it, whereas several decades ago it was hardly mentioned. To quote sex therapist Dr. Ruth: "I am not saying everybody is involved with oral sex, but . . . the one thing I can say with assurance to you is that there is nothing abnormal about it."

If you have religious scruples about oral sex, you might consult with your minister, priest, or rabbi. You may be surprised to find that the religious prohibitions you thought existed were misunderstandings on your part.

Needless to say, if either you or your partner has strong objections to this variation of lovemaking, do not feel any pressure to do something you would find disagreeable. If, on the other hand, you simply don't have much experience with oral lovemaking and you have some degree of concern or shyness, be aware that oral lovemaking is not rare and peculiar but quite common in our society.

Try giving yourself an opportunity to experiment, remembering how exciting those first sexual explorations were. It's fun to have new things to discover, especially now that you're over forty!

ENHANCING YOUR FEMALE
PARTNER'S SEXUAL
PLEASURE

The last three chapters concentrated on ways in which you and your partner can overcome and adapt to the sexual changes that you may experience after forty—in particular, the slowing of your erection responses and the decreased frequency of your desire for climax.

Your over-forty female partner, on the other hand, probably won't have the same decreased responses. In fact, most likely, she will be quite responsive to anything you can do to increase her enjoyment of lovemaking, to help her to have more satisfying climaxes, and even to please her at times when your own sexual responses may not be as strong as you might like.

As an older man, you may never have had the opportunity to actually learn the best ways to stimulate your partner and to bring her to a climax. In the past, sexual information wasn't as available, and many of us grew up thinking that whatever was going to happen during sex would happen during intercourse—and that if our partner didn't climax during intercourse, then maybe there was something wrong with *her.*

In fact, in your earliest years of sexual activity, you may not have even known that women were supposed to climax. One of my patients, Phil E., embarrassedly told me that the first time his wife climaxed he thought she was having a seizure. While this is an extreme example, many older men have told me they didn't really have any idea at all how a woman was supposed to respond—or how they could help her—when they had their first sexual encounters.

If you *were* aware that some women climaxed and your partner didn't, you may have thought that she was "frigid" or had some sexual problem. Your lack of knowledge was undoubtedly due more to the times than to lack of interest. You simply had never been taught about the ways that you could help a woman express and enjoy her sexuality. In fact, you probably were actively discouraged from learning by your parents and others.

Because of the negative attitudes toward sex with which couples now in their fifties and sixties were raised, many of us have never discussed intimate sexual issues with our partners. This lack of communication has made it difficult to learn from each other.

In your grandparents' time, the predominant feeling was that "nice women" were *not* supposed to respond sexually. If a woman assumed an active role during lovemaking or even became sexually aroused, it was actually seen as a sign that she had loose morals.

The naturalness of female sexual response was eventually recognized, but it was still defined in male terms by male doctors. Thus, orgasm during intercourse—and during intercourse only— was still felt to be the only normal way for a woman to climax until the scientific studies of Kinsey and Masters and Johnson appeared in the 1950s and '60s.. Before their conclusions were published, a woman who climaxed from clitoral stimulation was considered to be sexually immature.

With these studies of actual sexual response, it became clear that *most* women climax primarily or most readily with direct clitoral stimulation rather than during intercourse. Reports indicated that these women find that vaginal intercourse feels close, satisfying, and arousing, that they enjoy the feeling of having their partner's penis inside them, but that it's not the same kind of feeling that builds to climax for them. They simply require more direct oral or manual stimulation of their clitoris in order to climax. There's nothing wrong with them; it's just the way women's bodies are built and the way their sexual responses naturally are.

AN ERECTION ISN'T ALWAYS REQUIRED TO SATISFY YOUR PARTNER

The advantage for you as an older man in the way that women.climax is that it isn't necessary for you to have an erection every time you want to make love or every time you want to satisfy a woman.

Fred P., one of my patients in his late fifties, told me how pressured he felt to perform sexually if his wife felt like making love but he wasn't up to it. "I know there are times when she really expects us to make love, but I'm preoccupied and pooped and don't know if I can get it up—so I try to avoid the whole situation."

Many older men have felt like this at times. When you do, it's important to realize that there are other ways you can satisfy your partner, please her greatly, and enjoy yourself sexually without having to get an erection and without climaxing yourself.

Most older men have had some experience with helping a partner to climax by hand stimulation. However, sometimes either the

man or his partner may be self-conscious about manual stimulation, worrying that it's abnormal and that the only "normal" sex
is intercourse.

On the contrary, as we have already pointed out, clitoral stimulation is the natural way for most women to climax. Almost all
women, for example, stimulate their clitorises when masturbating,
while only 5 to 10 percent also insert objects in their vaginas. It's
clear that women, who are the best judges of what feels good to
themselves, find clitoral stimulation to be what produces orgasm
for them.

ORAL LOVEMAKING:
AN EXCITING ALTERNATIVE

In addition to manual stimulation, which you're probably already
familiar with, you both may very much enjoy the variation of using your mouth to stimulate her clitoris and genital area. Most
women find this kind of lovemaking, called *cunnilingus*, to be *extremely* pleasurable as well as warm, loving, and intimate. It also
provides something that couples who've been together for many
years need very much in their lovemaking—variety.

The soft caressing of the clitoris and vaginal lips is very sexually stimulating for women of all ages, and most women climax
more readily with cunnilingus than with intercourse. In fact, many
women who cannot climax with intercourse at all do so readily
with oral stimulation.

Using cunnilingus can relieve a lot of pressure to perform and
to get an erection when you just aren't able to. Once you've helped
your partner to climax with oral stimulation, you can feel confident that she feels both sexually satisfied and secure that you care

for her, and she will most likely be content to wait for intercourse until another time when you are ready. Moreover, this is an alternative lovemaking technique that you will greatly enjoy yourself—it's not only sensuous and pleasurable; it can make you proud of your ability to give your partner satisfaction and to help her climax.

Even if you are planning on intercourse, you can use cunnilingus either before or after intercourse to help your partner climax more readily, or just to help her get aroused. If you are using Viagra to help you get erect, you can use cunnilingus to stimulate your partner while you're waiting for the Viagra to kick in. It will certainly make your partner less impatient with any wait for the medication to work, and it will also let her know that you are thinking of her pleasure too, and not just about your own erection.

Many men in our age group have had little experience with giving oral stimulation. Some of us inevitably have leftover inhibitions about it and are just not comfortable doing it with our wives or partners.

Conversely, most younger people in our society take oral stimulation for granted as a familiar accompaniment to making love and a way of expressing love for their partners. It certainly might be worthwhile investigating this form of lovemaking yourself if you haven't already done so, if only to discover whether you and your own partner would also enjoy it.

HOW WILL MY PARTNER REACT?

If you haven't used oral stimulation before, your partner might certainly be a little hesitant at first, but she will undoubtedly enjoy it once you begin. Most women achieve a high level of excitation with cunnilingus, and the gentleness and softness of having her clitoris and vaginal lips kissed, licked, and lightly pulled by your lips can help produce an intense orgasm.

It's possible that your partner would like to try cunnilingus but has been afraid to ask about it. She may be reluctant to seem too forward, or she may assume that it would not appeal to you. Remember that many women have been raised to feel that mouth-genital contact is dirty and forbidden. They have been admonished to not even look at their genitals or touch them. Therefore, they are often surprised to learn that men usually enjoy the intimacy of cunnilingus and, rather than being repelled, find it quite exciting.

In order to introduce oral lovemaking to your partner, you might try discussing it first. On the other hand, it might be best to embark on it in the heat of the moment, to avoid the possible embarrassment or apprehension a self-conscious discussion beforehand might inspire. Your instincts in this matter will be your best guide.

It's probably optimal to pick a time when your partner has just bathed, so she won't be worried about cleanliness or body odor. Bathing or showering together and washing each other just before lovemaking is also a sensuous way to establish a mood. Using a fragrant massage or lovemaking oil may also help set her mind at ease.

Your partner's vaginal fluid will probably have no more taste than the taste of saliva when you're kissing. In some cases, there may be a sexy, arousing odor. Any unusual, unpleasant odor that can't be eliminated by bathing would indicate a problem, and a visit to her gynecologist would then be in order to see if the cause can be identified and eliminated.

If you are concerned about the sanitary aspects of cunnilingus, keep in mind that unless your partner has a vaginal infection, there are almost certainly many more bacteria and other germs in your mouth than there are in her vagina.

How to Begin   As you start mutually caressing and are both becoming sexually excited, use your mouth to kiss and lick her along her thighs and abdomen. These are sensitive areas, and doing so will also help her get used to having your mouth near her genitals. Then gradually brush your lips through her pubic hair, while you use your hand to stimulate her clitoris.

Your partner may respond with movements or sounds to indicate that she's enjoying what you're doing. If you're not sure, continue to kiss and lick her inner thighs, the crease of her thigh, and her pubic hair in a teasing way. One older woman told me smilingly that she had been apprehensive about her husband trying cunnilingus until she saw how much fun he was having rubbing his nose in her pubic hair. "Then," she said, "I just laughed and relaxed."

If you can tell that she is accepting and enjoying your lovemaking, spread your partner's legs apart and continue using your mouth to stimulate her genitals. This will probably be easiest to do if you lie between her legs while she is on her back with her knees spread apart and bent. You may also want to experiment with other positions, such as positioning yourself alongside her with your knees at the level of her shoulders so she can touch your genitals while you lean over and use your mouth to caress her clitoris and vaginal lips.

With your partner's legs spread, you'll notice that between the heavier folds of skin that make up the outer lips of her vulva there are two inner flaps, called the minor or inner lips. The vaginal opening is between these inner lips. Where they come together at the top there is a small nubbin of soft tissue, about half the size of the last joint on your pinkie. This is her clitoris. It's the most sensitive sexual area for most women, and it usually enlarges and becomes somewhat erect when a woman is sexually excited.

Other especially sensitive sexual areas will be the inside of her vaginal lips and the area right around the opening of her vagina. Deep inside her vagina there aren't as many nerve endings. The inside of the vagina is therefore less sensitive, except for a particular area of sensitivity called the G-spot, which we will describe in the next chapter.

Spread your partner's inner lips with your fingers and let your tongue run softly up and down the length of them. Then gradually move up her vaginal lips, using stroking, swirling, and licking movements around her clitoris. Some women enjoy stimulation directly on the clitoris, while others find it's too sensitive and prefer circular movements around it. Gentle sucking movements can also be very arousing. There's no rule of thumb here. Ask your partner what feels best to her. She may be embarrassed or too shy to tell you what she likes if you don't ask.

If your partner has never experienced oral stimulation before, she may be a little apprehensive and stiff at first, wondering whether you are enjoying it. Reassure her and try to get her to relax and concentrate on the sensations you're creating for her. Tell her to think about what your tongue feels like and to concentrate on the warmth, smoothness, and liquidness of the sensations that she's getting, instead of worrying about you.

While you're stimulating her clitoris with your tongue, you can also stimulate the opening of her vagina with your fingertip, or even fully insert your fingers.

Will She Climax?   Don't expect your partner to climax the first time you try oral stimulation. She may not be able to relax enough, or she may feel too self-conscious.

On the other hand, she may be surprised to climax again and

again. An advantage of oral lovemaking is that you can keep the stimulation up indefinitely, until either of you gets tired. And even if she does climax, you can keep licking her clitoris so that she can continue to have more orgasms—or else let her rest briefly in between two or more distinct climaxes. Some women find that their clitoris gets too sensitive immediately after one climax to allow them to proceed immediately to another.

Talk with your partner afterward about what it felt like to her. It may be a little difficult for her to sort through her feelings upon experiencing a type of lovemaking that she may have once thought of as shocking or improper. It may actually be disconcerting to her to discover that it felt exciting, and it may be difficult to initially acknowledge, even to herself, that she really enjoyed it.

If either of you has reservations after this first experience, don't be discouraged. Give yourselves a chance to become more accustomed to cunnilingus and more comfortable with your own enjoyment of it. Of course, never insist that your partner do anything in lovemaking that she's completely opposed to.

We should mention here that you will undoubtedly enjoy performing oral stimulation yourself. After all, your tongue and lips are among your most erotic organs, and your partner's wetness and softness will feel very pleasant and sensual to them. You will also be excited by her arousal, proud of your ability to express your love in such a warm, intimate way, and of your ability to give your partner such intense feelings of pleasure.

CHAPTER 12

MORE WAYS TO PLEASE
A WOMAN SEXUALLY

I've noted that the primary focus of sexual sensitivity for your partner is the area around her clitoris and her inner vaginal lips. But there is another area inside her vagina that may be very sensitive as well: the G-spot, or Graffenberg spot, named after the gynecologist who first described it in the 1950s.

Your partner's G-spot is located on the upper wall of her vagina when she's lying on her back. It's about an inch and a half inside her vaginal opening and is approximately the size of a quarter. It tends to feel rough, like tightly packed goose bumps, and swells when it's stimulated.

Women vary a great deal in their degree of sensitivity to G-spot stimulation. If your partner is responsive to this kind of stimulation, you are in a position to give her an incredible amount of sexual pleasure.

HOW TO STIMULATE YOUR
PARTNER'S G-SPOT

Whenever trying out a new sexual technique, it's best to do it when the two of you are at leisure to make love and won't be disturbed. Some women get a feeling of needing to urinate when their G-spot is first stimulated, so it might be a good idea for your partner to empty her bladder completely before you begin.

Start by giving your partner a soft back massage to help her relax. Then gradually extend your caresses over her buttocks. Gently caress the back of her legs and slide your hand between them. With her legs spread, apply a little warmed lovemaking oil or other sexual lubricant to her genital area and vaginal opening, and caress her clitoris gently. With your palm down, next gently insert one or two fingers into her vagina. Try stimulating the front wall of her vagina, about three-quarters of an inch past the border of her pubic bone in front. This will be about an inch and a half to two inches inside. Because she's lying on her stomach, you'll be pressing down, as if you were pressing toward her belly button.

Slide your fingers forward and back or side to side, and have your partner tell you when you've hit the sensitive place. As I mentioned above, it will probably feel rough, like goose bumps, to you. You may find that it becomes spongy, firm, and swells in size as you continue to stimulate it, much like the erectile tissue in your penis.

Now that you've found the G-spot, kneel between your partner's legs and caress the spot with the fingers of one hand while simultaneously using the thumb of the other to gently stimulate her clitoris. She may be able to climax in this position, or you have the alternative of continuing in a different position.

If your partner turns over onto her back, you can stimulate her

G-spot either kneeling alongside her or lying between her legs. If you are lying between her legs insert two fingers into her vagina and press upward. Move your fingers front to back and side to side. Also, try brushing your thumb or your tongue softly over her clitoris at the same time. Oral stimulation of your partner's clitoris while your fingers are stimulating her G-spot internally can be a very exciting combination of sensations for her. Have her tell you what feels best.

If you are kneeling beside your partner, you can reach down and insert two fingers into her vagina while leaning over and sucking or licking one of her nipples to give her a double sensation. Remember that you must curl your finger back in and up toward her abdominal wall to hit her G-spot. Many women find this combination of nipple and G-spot stimulation especially enjoyable.

Some women say that their climax has a different feel to it when it comes as a result of G-spot stimulation as opposed to exclusive clitoral stimulation, that it's deeper, more internal. Indeed, if your partner climaxes from G-spot stimulation, you may feel her pushing down against the tips of your fingers inside her vagina, instead of, or in addition to, her muscles squeezing around her vaginal opening, which you usually feel when she climaxes from clitoral stimulation alone.

TRYING G-SPOT STIMULATION DURING INTERCOURSE

Once you and your partner have located her G-spot, try stimulating it during intercourse. It may be difficult for your penis to make contact with your partner's G-spot in the standard missionary position with her lying on her back, so take this opportunity to experiment with other positions.

One that seems to work very well is the "female superior" position, in which you lie on your back and your partner kneels over you, facing you. In this position she can probably move her body so that your penis, which is angled forward, can press against her G-spot. Another often successful position is "rear entry," with your penis entering her vagina from behind.

For some women, lying on their back with their legs all the way up on their partner's shoulders enables his penis to contact this most sensitive spot. It sounds acrobatic, but most women don't find it too difficult at all.

Remember that there are many different ways to enjoy sex and that there isn't any best or "normal" way. There is individual variation among women, and the G-spot is more sensitive for some than for others. Some women just don't respond strongly to this kind of stimulation, so it's important not to get too involved in trying for a particular type or intensity of sexual response and considering it the only desirable one.

Let the sensitive spot inside your partner's vagina be an additional toy that the two of you can play with. It can become a pleasurable way of varying your sexual repertoire that you can enjoy together indefinitely.

HELPING YOUR PARTNER HAVE
MORE THAN ONE CLIMAX

You and your partner have probably heard of multiple climaxes for women but may have never really tried to actually achieve them. If she usually has a single clear-cut orgasm, she may never have attempted to climax again after it. If the two of you experiment together, however, you may find that a woman's capacity for more than one climax can add another interesting variation to your lovemaking.

If you are trying to help your partner have multiple climaxes for the first time, the easiest way to begin is for you to stimulate her orally while lying between her legs. Then, while you're licking her clitoris, insert two of your fingers in her vagina to also gently stimulate her G-spot, as we have just described.

You're probably used to ceasing stimulation when your partner reaches her first major climax. This time, keep her clitoris pressed against your lips as she is climaxing and continue to gently stimulate it with your tongue. You may both be surprised to find that she climaxes a second time, and perhaps even a third or fourth, a few seconds apart. Each climax will be a separate peak, without the relaxation that usually occurs after her first climax. She may get tired or too sensitive to continue after several orgasms, but on another occasion she may be curious to see just how many times she can actually climax in a row.

One warning: Sometimes a woman's clitoris becomes exquisitely sensitive immediately after climaxing—so much so that she can't stand to have it touched. If this happens, you can still prolong her excitement by continuing to stimulate her G-spot internally with your fingers while you withdraw your lips from her clitoris. Then, after fifteen or twenty seconds, you can return to extremely gentle clitoral stimulation with your tongue, and gradually build the intensity to help her to climax again.

Don't worry if your partner doesn't climax a second time even with this additional stimulation. The intensity of her first climax may have been so strong that she simply doesn't need additional climaxes.

A VIBRATOR CAN BE
A WELCOME ADDITION

Men and women over fifty or so usually have little experience with sexual vibrators, which became popular as sexual toys long after most of our sexual training was completed. But vibrators, along with the other sexual suggestions in this book, can be worthy electives in your post-forty sexual education.

The vibrator/massager actually provides something new and different. Its rapid vibration applied to sexually sensitive areas provides a stimulation more intense than any that can be provided by simple movement of hand or tongue. Using a vibrator can help you give your female partner a new kind of intense sexual stimulation as well as provide variety and spice to your lovemaking. You can also be confident that at those times when you're unsure of your erection ability, you can provide pleasure for your partner in an interesting and different way.

There are three basic types of vibrators, all of which are hand held. The first two operate on electrical current and must be plugged into an outlet. The third is usually battery operated.

The first type, sometimes called a Swedish massager, is strapped to the back of your hand so that your fingers and palm pulsate with it. It provides a vibrating sensation through your hand to whatever part of your partner's body you touch. Some people find the sensation to be quite pleasurable, while others find that the vibrator numbs their hand after a while and becomes uncomfortable.

The second type of vibrator is held in your hand rather than strapped to it. It looks something like a compact kitchen mixer. Indeed, some of these vibrator/massagers are made by companies that also make kitchen blenders, such as Oster. This model comes with various small attachments, including cup and disc pieces you can use to stimulate various parts of your own or your partner's body. Women often enjoy having their clitoral area stimulated with a cup-shaped attachment or an attachment with a central ball. Men may enjoy the cup shape over the tip of their penis.

The third type of vibrator is usually battery operated. It's cylindrical and tapered and shaped approximately like a penis. Most often used to stimulate the clitoral area, it sometimes is also inserted into the vagina. Although most women climax primarily with clitoral stimulation, many report that they enjoy the feeling of having the vibrator in their vagina to squeeze on while they're climaxing.

Vibrators are sold in drugstores, department stores, medical supply stores, in catalogues, and on the Internet. They are often sold as foot, hand, or back massagers, and some buyers actually use them for this purpose.

A caveat concerning battery-operated models: They sometimes turn out to be flimsy in construction, so it's best to make any purchase through a reputable source. It's also important to always make sure your vibrator is clean before use.

Following are some suggestions for stimulating your partner with the cylindrical, tapered, penis-shaped vibrator. You can adapt these suggestions to the other two types equally effectively in slightly different ways.

If your partner is lying on her stomach, begin by using the vibrator to give her a relaxing back massage. Then spread her legs gently with your hand and apply a small amount of lovemaking oil or other lubricant to her vaginal area and clitoris. Lubricate the vibrator, as well.

It's pleasurable at all stages to combine vibrator stimulation with your own caresses, using your hands, mouth, and penis.

While you slide the vibrator up your partner's inner thighs and approach her vulva in a teasing fashion, gently caress her back and buttocks with your other hand. Then run the length of the vibrator gently down the crease of her buttocks. If the vibrator and her vaginal area are both well lubricated, the vibrator will slip almost effortlessly between her vaginal lips. One of my patients told me that the first time she felt a vibrator in her vaginal area she couldn't believe how intense the sensation was.

Feel with your fingertip for the opening of her vagina. Then very gradually insert the tip of the vibrator. Slowly, and very gently, continue to slide the vibrator in as you would your penis. Remember, your partner must tell you if it's uncomfortable in any way.

Continue to hold the vibrator in her vagina with one hand. Then with the other hand gently caress her clitoris and vulval lips while the vibrator rests against your fingers. It will feel to her as if your fingers, too, are vibrating, and this will be very stimulating. Ask her at all stages to tell you what feels comfortable, and what degree of pressure she enjoys.

With the vibrator inserted, the stimulation will become even more intense to her. You can add to it by gently sliding the vibrator back out about an inch and then in again in gentle thrusts. If your partner enjoys that, you can add to her sensation by gently moving the vibrator from side to side—especially if you simultaneously stimulate her clitoris with your free hand. If you have previously located her G-spot, try to stimulate it with the tip of the vibrator. Don't be surprised if she climaxes at this time.

Now let your partner turn over on her back. Slide the vibrator gently up and down her abdomen and around her pubic area. Gently caress one of her breasts with your hand or tongue while you gradually slide the vibrator down past your partner's abdomen and slip it between her legs. Gently slide it forward and back against her vaginal lips while you lick her nipples or caress them with your fingers. She'll enjoy the combination of feelings.

Touch the area around her clitoris softly with the tip of the vibrator, while sliding the fingers of your other hand into her vagina. If you press the vibrator against that hand, your fingers inside her vagina will vibrate, and your partner will receive an interesting and wildly arousing variety of sensations.

Then slide the vibrator gradually into her vaginal opening. Withdraw it an inch or so and gently slide it back in with a soft, thrusting movement. Your partner can have the most exquisite arousal if you manually stimulate her clitoris or lick it at the same time.

Proceed to intercourse at this point, if you wish. Certain positions will even enable you to continue to use the vibrator to stimulate your partner's clitoris while you're inside her. Have her lie on her side, for example, with her back toward you, while you lie on your side behind her. Then come into her vagina from behind. You can easily reach across her abdomen and stimulate her clitoris with the vibrator while your penis is inside her. Use your imagination to devise other ways. Your partner will have the extraordinary feeling of your penis inside her while her clitoris is simultaneously receiving this intense stimulation from the vibrator, and your penis will also feel the vibration through her vaginal walls.

When used in this way, a vibrator can add dimension and variety to your lovemaking. Many people, however, feel that while the physical sensation produced by the vibrator is intense, there is also a loss of intimacy, resulting in sex that is less emotionally satisfying than that which comes from direct hand-to-body or mouth-to-body contact.

It's also extremely important not to use the vibrator too frequently. If your partner uses a vibrator regularly in order to climax, she may become insensitive to other forms of stimulation.

The vibrator stimulation is so intense that it's hard for a finger or tongue to compete with it. She can then become dependent on the vibrator in order to climax and may no longer respond to manual or oral stimulation—or even to intercourse—as intensely as she did before. It's therefore wise to keep a vibrator as an occasional plaything only, in which case it will be an interesting variation in your lovemaking.

AN IMPORTANT REVIEW ABOUT YOUR PARTNER'S CLIMAXES

There are important points I'd like to make about a woman's sexual responses.

Your Partner Doesn't Need to Climax During Intercourse For most women, intercourse is simply not the best way of producing the stimulation required for orgasm. Although they enjoy the intimacy of intercourse, it just doesn't provide the direct stimulation that enables them to climax.

I have often come across women in my practice who were very sexually responsive, easily aroused, desirous of sex, and who climaxed easily with oral or manual stimulation of the clitoris, but who complained that they were "frigid." It would turn out that they defined themselves as frigid because they didn't climax during intercourse. We now know that such women are normal and sexually responsive, and that most women respond the same way: They climax more readily, or even *exclusively*, with direct clitoral stimulation.

Your Partner Doesn't Need to Climax at the Same Time You Do Another myth that can interfere with your sexual pleasure is the idea that simultaneous orgasms are the best and most satisfy-ing. Some women may indeed prefer this, but it's not a standard that everybody desires or must try to achieve. In fact, many cou-ples feel that it's more pleasurable to climax one at a time, so that each can concentrate while climaxing and the other can have the enjoyment of watching as well. Remember that a woman can cli-max before, during, or after intercourse—or at all three times, if she likes.

Your Partner Doesn't Have to Have Multiple Orgasms   Earlier in this chapter we described how you may be able to help your partner have multiple climaxes. But also remember that there isn't anything wrong with her if she doesn't. Many women experience an extremely satisfying single orgasm, totally complete in itself. Other women vary, sometimes climaxing singly, other times mul-tiply. Neither experience is any better, more sexual, or more suc-cessful than the other.

Your Partner Doesn't Need to Climax Every Time You Make Love   There may be times when your partner just doesn't feel the need to climax in a particular lovemaking episode. It may be be-cause she is tired, not feeling quite right, or just feeling less re-sponsive for no particular reason. Leave yourselves open to enjoy whatever happens in your lovemaking without pushing yourselves to meet standards of performance. There may be times when you may not have the need to climax but she may have an orgasm, or vice versa. As long as each of you is enjoying the lovemaking and neither of you is feeling taken advantage of, either of these op-tions is perfectly all right. It's only a problem if one or the other of you is *consistently* unable to climax.

CHAPTER 13

PROLONGING YOUR LOVEMAKING FOR HOURS

Men over forty have the advantage of not needing to climax every time they make love. This gives them considerably more flexibility in their sexual relations than they had when they were younger. Now that you're over forty, you can use this flexibility to build your sexual tension or to extend your lovemaking over an entire day or even a weekend.

In this chapter I'll describe how slow, unpressured lovemaking can allow you to be sexually stimulated and intermittently erect all day long—instead of having a disappointing and embarrassing loss of sexual desire and ability after an initial sexual encounter.

You will also learn other ways to turn your ability to enjoy sex without climaxing into an advantage, and how you can use brief lovemaking as an "appetizer" when you're short on time—in anticipation of more extensive love play later on.

PROLONGING YOUR LOVEMAKING
FOR SPECIAL OCCASIONS

You and your partner may be planning a romantic day of lovemaking to celebrate an anniversary, a weekend in the country, or just a rainy Sunday. As a man over forty or fifty, however, you may be concerned that after you've made love once, it may take you quite a while until you feel like making love a second time—and longer still until you can get another erection. You'll be glad to know how easy it can be to get around this problem, and enjoy doing it.

You can probably remember times when you started out feeling that you wanted to make love all day but found that once you climaxed the first time your sexual drive and interest disappeared. You and your partner may have felt disappointed at having your romantic day cut short, and you may have felt somewhat foolish and embarrassed, having talked about how you would like to make love "all day long."

There is an easy way to avoid this. The falloff in sexual drive doesn't come from making love; it comes from climaxing. Now that you're older, it will take longer than it did ten, twenty, or thirty years ago to feel like lovemaking again after you've had a climax.

But there is a good-news side to this, too. You can take advantage of another of the changes of aging—your increased ability to enjoy sex without ejaculating—to prolong your lovemaking in a delightful way and to increase your sexual tension at the same time. In many cases, you really can make love "all day long."

ENJOY SLOW, UNPRESSURED LOVEMAKING

Let me describe how you *could* make love all day for a special occasion!

At your first encounter of the day, start off with some mutual caressing to help you get hard and your partner lubricated. As you will be engaged in a lot of sexual activity today, a sexual lubricant may be helpful in keeping either of you from getting sore. Proceed to intercourse when you're ready, using any position that you both enjoy and that gives you good control over your ejaculation. Penetrate slowly and leisurely, concentrating on the feeling of your penis inside your partner's vagina.

Take your time kissing and caressing while continuing your slow, luxuriating intercourse. Then, before you get close to climaxing, withdraw but continue caressing. If your erection has gone down, your partner can help you get hard again.

After taking time to relax and caress, return again to slow-paced intercourse. Use a different position if you desire. Again, remember not to push rapidly for climax but rather enjoy the sensual experience. If, for instance, you have inserted your penis into your partner's vagina from behind, with the two of you lying on your sides in a spoon position, give her a soft back massage while you continue to gently move your penis in and out. You can stop thrusting for a while and then restart—or even let your erection go down, withdraw, and return to kissing and caressing.

Most women are able to climax more than once without having their sex drive diminish. Your partner may climax anytime during this first session of lovemaking, or else allow her sexual tension to build along with yours until later in the day.

YOU MAY FEEL STIMULATED ALL DAY

The two of you can then take a break and go to lunch, take a walk, or enjoy some other activity. You'll discover that since you've had so much sexual stimulation without ejaculation, instead of feeling the loss of interest that you ordinarily feel after sex, you will continue to enjoy the sensation of being sexually aroused throughout your other activities. You may both continue to have thoughts and fantasies about sex and feel anxious to get back to another lovemaking session in the afternoon.

When you return to continue your celebration, your partner can help you to get erect again, and you can also resume caressing her. The two of you may alternate manual with oral petting to excite each other and have relaxed episodes of intercourse.

After another hour or more of leisurely lovemaking in the afternoon, you can break for another activity and take up lovemaking once more in the evening. Or you can finish your lovemaking by climaxing at any time.

After holding off from climaxing over a long period of time, you may occasionally find that you are unable to come when you finally want to. If so, don't worry about it. Just wait until the next sexual opportunity and let yourself climax easily the first time.

This kind of prolonged lovemaking without climaxing has wonderful advantages for those occasions when you have all the time in the world. It allows a slow, leisurely, and especially tender sharing.

Prolonged lovemaking isn't always necessary, though. Many times, sex will be complete in a single episode, and that's perfectly all right. But for those times when you know that there will be many sexual opportunities during a day or weekend, and you would like to make love more than once, prolonged lovemaking without climaxing can greatly increase your pleasure.

If you are using Viagra to enable or enhance your erection, there are a couple of strategies that you can use to have it better fit into your schedule. In the first place, while Viagra takes awhile to be effective, its effect usually lasts for several hours anyway, so if your lovemaking won't be too extended, it may last long enough without any help.

If you wish it to last longer you might consider a different strategy: While ordinarily you probably try to take it on an empty stomach so that the onset will be more rapid, now your goal is different. If you take it *after* a meal the onset will be slower but the duration will be longer. You may need to take a somewhat larger dose if you are taking Viagra after a meal than you ordinarily take in order to achieve the same blood levels. Discuss this with your doctor.

A third choice, which you also should discuss with your doctor, would be to take Viagra more than once during the day. Viagra is only recommended for once a day on the package insert, but there is no obvious reason why taking it twice in a day on occasion would cause any difficulty, especially if you are taking one of the lower dosages. Again, ask your doctor who knows your individual medical condition.

THE APPETIZER: WHEN THERE ISN'T TIME FOR MORE

Your advantage of not needing to climax every time can also give you a lot more flexibility on those occasions when you and your partner are both sexually excited and want to make love but you have only a few minutes for lovemaking. You may have to get dressed soon to go out for dinner or to go to work. You may already be dressed. Company may be expected at any moment, or an appointment may have to be kept. It may even be late at night, and you have to arise early in the morning. You may feel like making love but know that you don't have time for full, extended lovemaking.

Let's assume that the two of you have just showered and have company arriving in forty-five minutes. Showering together has gotten you both sexually interested, but you must dress and finish preparing for your guests. You realize that the extended lovemaking session you both want must be postponed until after the company leaves. This is a good time for a little "warm-up."

Ask your partner if she would like to "play" a little before you get dressed. If she's receptive, as you caress and stroke each other, you will probably both become aroused. Your partner can help you get fully erect. Some oral stimulation may be especially helpful to you at a time like this—and you can use it as well to help your partner become rapidly lubricated. Applying a sexual lubricant to your penis and to her vagina will also help you achieve an easy entry.

When you are fairly hard and well lubricated, you can slide into your partner for a little sexual appetizer and promise of things to come. *Don't* rush, and *don't* try to climax. Make some nice, gentle thrusts and press yourself fully inside her.

This little appetizer can be as brief as four or five strokes or as long as four or five minutes before you withdraw without climaxing. It's a wonderful way of letting each other know how much you care about each other. And, during dinner, you can both be thinking about how much you'll enjoy "dessert."

You can even try a sexual appetizer when you're both fully dressed, though it will require you to be a little more imaginative and uninhibited. Let's say that this time you only have *fifteen* minutes until the guests are due to arrive, and you don't have time to get fully undressed and dressed again. On the other hand, you're both feeling sexy and would like a little love play.

Your partner can open your pants and caress your penis manually or orally to help you get hard. If she is wearing a skirt, put your hand under it and caress her genital area to help her lubricate while she's caressing you. A small amount of sexual lubricant carefully applied so as not to get any on her clothing will be very helpful.

When you're erect and she's lubricated, she can simply slip down her panties or panty hose and lean over a counter, a bed, or the dining-room table. Pull her skirt up over her buttocks from behind and, with you standing behind her, let her guide your penis into her vagina. You will both find it very exciting when you caress her buttocks and genitals with her dress pulled up or her slacks pulled down. If necessary, you both can be fully dressed again in seconds! And, who knows, the guests may be late!

Again, just a few strokes or a few minutes of lovemaking in a situation like this will leave you both feeling very daring, sexually stimulated, and looking forward to lovemaking later. The experience of brief intercourse without orgasm is a wonderful way of showing your desire for each other when time is limited. You may occasionally have difficulty getting hard because you're worried that the time is short. Trying to get an erection quickly can cause occasional problems for anyone. If you do have difficulty, don't be concerned. Just enjoy the fun and warmth of caressing each other sexually, and try again at another time.

Half of a Viagra may help assure erection at a pressured time like this, but you will need to take it a little in advance. Even on an empty stomach it will take at least ten to twenty minutes to work.

MIDDLE-OF-THE-NIGHT, HALF-ASLEEP PLAY

The ability to make love without needing to climax can be enjoyed at those times when you're just dozing off or when you wake up warm and cuddly in the middle of the night or in the morning.

You may both be half asleep and not up to fully energetic love-making, but you may also feel sensual, a little excited, and open to a little sexual play. It is best to have discussed the possibility of this kind of sexual adventure in advance so it won't come as a surprise to your partner when she's half asleep.

Let's say, for example, your partner is tired and you're giving her a back rub to help her relax before sleep. As she starts dozing off, slide one of your massaging hands down between her legs and gradually and gently caress her vulva and help her lubricate without fully waking her. Continue to rub her back with the other hand. Go back and forth for a while, rubbing her back, then returning to her vulva, and adding a little lubricant so that she will be quite wet. You will likely be partially erect from stimulating her, and then, by gently rubbing your penis against her thigh, you may become fully hard.

Put a little lubrication on your own penis, spread her legs, and slip gently inside her while she continues to lie facedown, half dozing. She need not fully awaken, but it will help if she tilts her pelvis up toward you or if you slip a pillow under her to facilitate penetration.

After thrusting softly for a minute or two, you can then both roll over on your sides, with your penis still inside her vagina from behind. After a few more gentle thrusts, you can both fall asleep with you still inside her, a very tender and romantic way of living out a sexual fantasy.

Another scenario: You awaken in the early-morning hours with an erection. If your partner is sleeping with her back toward you, you can gently stroke her vaginal area from behind to see if she is receptive. If she seems to enjoy what you're doing, lubricate her vaginal area with a lubricant that you keep by the bedside, making sure to warm it briefly in your hand first.

Then gently slip your penis inside her. If you're both three-quarters asleep, you can make just a few thrusting movements and fall back asleep. Your penis will, of course, slip out as your erection goes down, but you will both reawaken later in the morning feeling terrific and loved. You can finish your lovemaking when you're fully awake, or else save it for evening.

Make sure you let your partner know how much you appreciate her loving cooperation and how wonderful it makes you feel to know that you can initiate love play at almost any time and to know that in most cases she will be lovingly receptive. Remember that these little nighttime or morning play sessions don't have to go anywhere. You don't have to climax during them. They are just a sign of your love and affection for each other.

BUILDING SEXUAL TENSION

A final benefit of lovemaking without climaxing is that it can be used to greatly increase your level of sexual tension. If you become sexually aroused two or three times in the course of a day from manual or oral stimulation of your penis, as well as intercourse, and if you continue again the next day with more of the same without climaxing, you may start to feel an increased sense of sexual urgency and desire that you may not have experienced for a long time. You may find yourself thinking more sexually, feeling more sensitivity from your penis, and even becoming aroused and erect more easily. Even though repeated sexual arousal throughout the day may not be practical on a regular basis, it's a real delight on occasion.

CHAPTER 14

SIMPLE EXERCISES TO STRENGTHEN YOUR SEXUAL MUSCLES

I've often been asked whether there are exercises that can help improve sexual functioning and sexual response. There are, and they can be used by both men and women to strengthen their sexual muscles and improve their responses. Called Kegel exercises, they can be especially important for older men and women, to prevent the loss of pelvic muscle tone that might otherwise come with aging.

As a woman over forty, you may have noticed that the muscles around your vagina have lost some of their tone and are looser than they used to be, especially if you have had several children. This may give you and your partner less friction and, consequently, less intensity during intercourse.

Doing Kegel exercises can help you tighten these muscles yourself without surgery. Moreover, Kegels can improve your vaginal tone and enable you to climax more easily, with more intense orgasms. Your strengthened vaginal muscles will also provide more friction during intercourse and allow you to squeeze your partner's penis more tightly. This may be especially important if his erection is not quite fully firm at first, which is not uncommon for older men.

Many men also feel that the Kegel exercises help them sexually. Some of my male patients say the exercises give them more control over premature ejaculation, help them have stronger, more pleasurable orgasms, and help with erection problems.

HOW A WOMAN CAN STRENGTHEN HER SEXUAL MUSCLES

Your sexual muscle is the pubococcygeus, often called the PC muscle. It surrounds the opening to your vagina and extends from your pubic bone to your tailbone, or coccyx.

For many women the PC muscle loses its tone and tightness with age, and especially after childbirth. If the problem becomes severe, these vaginal muscles can be repaired and tightened surgically. In most cases, however, this isn't necessary. You can perform a simple set of exercises to tighten and tone your PC muscles yourself.

These exercises were developed several decades ago by Dr. Arnold Kegel, who originally used them to help women tighten their vaginas and overcome urinary stress incontinence after childbirth.

The easiest way for a woman to locate her PC muscle is to discover it during urination. While urinating, try stopping and starting the urine flow with your legs spread wide apart. The muscle that you squeeze to stop the flow is your PC muscle. Check by inserting the tip of your finger into your vagina and contracting your muscle just the way you did to stop urinating. If you have any muscle tone, you should notice a slight tightening of the vagina around your finger.

When you have a clear idea of what the contractions feel like, allow yourself a few minutes to practice them. While lying comfortably on your bed, tighten and then release the muscle ten times. Gradually increase this from day to day until you are doing fifty contractions each day.

Once you have developed some ease with these exercises, you can do them at any time—while you're driving your car, sitting at your desk, or talking on the telephone—and no one else will ever know what you're doing.

Once you can do fifty contractions fairly easily, you can begin some variations: First, quickly contract or tighten the muscle, then very gradually relax it. Do ten of these variations and add them in as part of your usual fifty per day.

The second series of variations is a fast tightening followed by a fast relaxation. This is a speeded-up version of what you were doing all along. Again, include this variation among the fifty that you are doing daily.

The third variation is to tighten very, very slowly, being aware of how deep in the vagina you can feel the contraction. When you feel your entire pelvic area totally tensed, quickly relax. This may take some practice, so don't become discouraged if you have some difficulty feeling it.

After you've built up your strength so that you can do these exercises easily and when you can feel a definite squeeze on your finger when you contract your muscle, you can drop down to doing only twenty per day. You will have developed good tone and control at this point, so you will just be maintaining your muscle strength. Some women, however, continue to do fifty or more squeezes a day, either because it increases their sexual awareness or because they wish to build their ability to grip their partner's penis during intercourse.

Some women report that they climax more readily as they develop more strength in their PC muscles. Other women find that their enjoyment of their orgasm is greater because their contractions are more intense. As we noted before, strengthening your PC muscle can also increase your partner's enjoyment, since you can readily squeeze to stimulate his penis during intercourse. He will also be able to feel your more intense contractions during orgasm.

Of equal importance: PC exercises are a significant way for you to continue to maintain and care for your sexual system as you age. Maintaining the PC muscle is not only a daily exercise of your sexual system; it's also an investment in sexual enjoyment.

HOW MEN CAN STRENGTHEN THEIR OWN SEXUAL MUSCLES

Men, too, can benefit greatly from doing Kegel exercises. Your penis gets erect not from tightening a muscle but because it fills with blood. There aren't any significant muscles in the penis itself, but the entire base of the penis, which is inside your body, is surrounded by your pelvic muscles. The sexual benefits of strengthening the male PC muscle have not been scientifically proven, but there is accumulating empirical evidence that it helps in a number of ways.

In the first place, strengthening and exercising the pelvic muscles surrounding the base of your penis will help to increase the blood supply to those muscles and to the entire pelvic area, including the penis. This can improve the circulation of blood in the penis and, theoretically, improve erections in that way.

Second, if not exercised, the PC muscle tends to atrophy somewhat with age. Since one of the features of orgasm is the rhythmic contraction of this muscle, its atrophy means decreased sensation from orgasm.

Thus, exercising your PC muscle and strengthening it may give you stronger, more pleasurable orgasms. It may also help you to develop better control over your ejaculation as you become more consciously aware of your sexual response. With practice, men can learn to either firmly contract or consciously relax this muscle, so that they can voluntarily delay the onset of ejaculation.

A number of patients over forty have told me that doing Kegel exercises has also improved their prostate function. In fact, several have said that their bouts with chronic prostatitis, which had previously required frequent or continuous antibiotic therapy, had subsided completely after several months of doing Kegel exercises. Urologists I have checked with don't know of any studies that prove Kegel exercises actually help prostatitis, but since contractions of the PC muscle may help the prostate to drain and may increase blood circulation in the area of the gland, it's certainly possible that these exercises might be beneficial. At any rate, they are something very simple that you can do yourself that might help and won't be of any harm.

You can locate your PC muscle the same way we directed women to locate theirs earlier in the chapter. Try stopping and starting the flow of urine while you're urinating. Or else, pretend that you're trying to hold in a bowel movement. The muscles you squeeze to do this are the pelvic muscles you're looking for.

Once you've located the muscles, try squeezing and releasing them fifteen times twice a day. Gradually increase the number of contractions from day to day, until you're doing fifty at a time.

At this point you can add a variation. Contract your pelvic muscles and hold them for three seconds before you relax. Try to work up to doing fifty of these longer Kegel exercises twice a day. You can alternate a series of these with the regular short Kegels.

It may take a month until you begin to feel sexual benefits from these exercises, but you probably should continue them for at least six weeks to see if they will be helpful for you.

MASTURBATION WHEN YOU ARE WITHOUT A PARTNER

Older men, and older women alike, may find themselves without sexual partners at times due to divorce, death, or illness of a partner, or temporary separation. At times like this, self-stimulation (or masturbation), as a way of dealing with your normal sexual desire, is a common, sensible solution. It also may be thought of as an important sexual exercise to keep yourself ready for the possibility of resuming sexual relations sometime in the future.

Many of us who are over fifty and sixty received our ideas about masturbation from parents with prejudices left over from the Victorian era. It's difficult now, in retrospect, to imagine how such a safe, harmless practice could arouse such phobias. After all, when you pleasure yourself, no one becomes pregnant, is molested, catches a venereal disease, or is harmed in any way.

Almost all adolescent boys and about two-thirds of adolescent girls masturbate. The high frequency of masturbation during adolescence doesn't mean that masturbation is a particularly adolescent activity. It merely reflects the fact that adolescents have a high sex drive and don't have readily available sexual partners. Masturbation resumes or continues, for most men and women, at other times in their lives when they don't have a regular partner. It doesn't represent sexual immaturity or perversion. It just represents not having someone else to have sex with.

If you're over forty, continuing some form of sexual activity is important as a way of keeping your sexual organs and sexual physiology healthy and functioning. If you go for a long time without using your body in a sexual way, resuming sex may become much more difficult.

If, for example, a man has been having regular erections with masturbation, it will be much easier for him to function in a sexual situation than if he had not had any erections for years. Similarly, for an older woman, lack of regular arousal for a long period of time may worsen vaginal atrophy and make it more difficult for the vagina to lubricate and to stretch to accommodate a penis during intercourse. Masturbation is a good way of keeping sexual function intact during that time when a partner is unavailable.

Masturbation, however, cannot make up for the lack of a sexual partner, and despite the physical benefits, it's natural to have some feelings of being unfulfilled. There are, however, some things that you can do to make masturbation more pleasurable for yourself.

To start off with, allow yourself plenty of time. Pleasuring yourself isn't something to just rush through and get out of the way. Prepare some atmosphere: candlelight, music perhaps, and ensure privacy by unplugging your telephone.

Fantasy, common for both men and women during masturbation, will enable you to feel more sexual and aroused. You can help yourself fantasize by reading sexually oriented books or watching erotic videotapes.

Lubricants will help to simulate the wetness of sexual intercourse. They also prevent irritation and make masturbation more comfortable and pleasant.

A vibrator can provide variety as well as extra stimulation. A woman can use it on her clitoris or a man on the head of his penis. Some women enjoy the pulsating quality of a stream of water from their shower attachment while they lie in the tub.

Use your imagination so that masturbation can provide you pleasure and sexual relief when your partner is not available and help to keep your sexual mechanism functioning well.

PART

4

SEX AND YOUR HEALTH
AFTER FORTY

CHAPTER 15

SATISFYING SEX IN SPITE
OF ARTHRITIS AND
LOWER-BACK PAIN

More people in this country are affected by arthritis than by any other disease, and most of these people are over forty.

Unfortunately, if you have arthritis, you know that the stiffness, pain, fatigue, and limitation of motion that too often accompany this illness can unquestionably affect your sexual life, as can lower-back pain, which also afflicts many older people. This chapter will offer ways that you and your partner can adapt and adjust to these problems so you can continue to enjoy a full sex life together.

Arthritis limits physical activity—all kinds of physical activity. If you have arthritis, you may lose the ease and comfort of movement that you once had. Mobility in some of your joints may be lost completely, as may the dexterity of the fine movements of your hands. Unfortunately, in addition to limiting other *physical* activity, the discomfort of arthritis can markedly limit a person's *sexual* activity.

I remember fifty-year-old Rebecca W. telling me, "Sometimes the pain was excruciating when I tried to spread my legs for intercourse. It didn't happen every time, but after a while I became afraid to try. It's hard to feel sexy when you're waiting for a stab of pain." I couldn't argue with that, but I was able to show her how to enjoy sex again—in ways I'll discuss later in this chapter.

The pain of arthritis can influence your sexual life in two ways. First, it may have a direct effect: It may make it difficult to reach orgasm if, for instance, the position that you're using for lovemaking causes your hip to hurt, or if you are afraid that pain may start. Second, there may be an indirect effect: Chronic pain anywhere in your body can decrease your sexual drive and distract you during lovemaking, even if the joint involved has nothing to do with the lovemaking itself.

It's not only the pain and stiffness of arthritis that can limit your sexual activity. You may also inhibit yourself due to lack of confidence about your physical appearance, since arthritis may cause swelling and deformity in some of your joints.

The role you take in sex can also influence your feelings. Men who are used to being the more active partner in lovemaking may feel that they're giving up their masculine role if they have to limit their movements and let their partners take over the more active role.

YOUR PARTNER MAY HOLD BACK, TOO

If your partner knows that you have pain and discomfort during sex, he or she may avoid suggesting lovemaking altogether rather than cause you discomfort, and may even feel guilty and selfish about suggesting it knowing it may be uncomfortable for you.

THE MANY BENEFITS OF STAYING SEXUALLY ACTIVE

It's extraordinarily important to keep a positive attitude toward lovemaking and to stay as sexually active as you can, even with arthritis. Successful lovemaking will improve your image of yourself and increase your self-esteem. It's a wonderfully effective way to restore your self-confidence in your physical self and reinforce your feeling of masculinity or femininity.

Sex may relieve pain, too. Some people experience pain *relief* for up to six to eight hours after sexual relations. It is thought that this may be due to the body's release of endorphins, its internal pain relievers, during sexual stimulation and especially during orgasm.

You and your partner can take a number of basic steps to help you overcome some of the sexual problems caused by arthritis. The steps may be simple, but they can be very important. Some may seem unromantic and unspontaneous to you, but your lovemaking will probably be more enjoyable if it's planned but pain-free than it will be if it's spontaneous but uncomfortable.

STEP 1: WORK WITH YOUR PARTNER ON HOW YOU BOTH CAN ADAPT TO YOUR PHYSICAL LIMITATIONS

Let your partner know what touches are uncomfortable or painful. Guide your partner's hand with yours to show him or her which tender areas need to be avoided. Also show your partner how he or she can stimulate you without causing you pain.

You may not have talked about things like this in specific ways before, but doing so now can be crucial. Your partner will have less worry about causing you pain while caressing you if you've explained your sensitive areas in advance. And you will be better able to relax and enjoy lovemaking as well if you know that he or she is aware of your particularly painful points and will try to avoid them.

STEP 2: DEVELOP A CLEAR SIGNAL TO COMMUNICATE DISCOMFORT

Developing a clear signal in advance will allow you to let your partner know quickly and easily if lovemaking becomes uncomfortable for you. A tap on the shoulder, for instance, may be much less disruptive to the lovemaking mood than saying "Ouch!" or "Stop!"

STEP 3: CHOOSE THE BEST TIME OF DAY FOR YOU

Different types of arthritis have different patterns of discomfort throughout the day. If, for example, you have rheumatoid arthritis, you may feel particularly stiff in the morning and better later in the day. If, on the other hand, you have osteoarthritis, you may feel worse in the evening and better in the morning. Choose your best time of day for making love. Try to adapt your lovemaking schedule to your own body's needs. For instance, if you feel stiff in the morning, but tired in the evening, try to make love in the afternoon whenever possible. Take advantage of the time after you feel loosened up but before you become fatigued.

STEP 4: PLAN AROUND YOUR
MEDICATION SCHEDULE

Some people with arthritis or back pain take pain medication or anti-inflammatory medication on a regular schedule. If you do, try to plan your lovemaking around it. You probably know approximately how quickly your medication takes effect, so try for that period when the medication is at peak effectiveness. On the other hand, if your medication sedates you or dulls your sensitivity, you might wish to wait until the sedation passes or to discuss a change in your medication with your physician.

STEP 5: MAKE THE MOST OF
YOUR MEDICATION OPTIONS

If you have tried several different medications and none has worked the way you want it to, don't give up! Check with your doctor regularly as newer treatments with more efficacy and fewer side effects continue to become available.

Confide in your doctor if a particular joint, such as your hip, knee, or back, interferes with your sexual activity. Specific physical therapy for that joint might make a difference, while a local cortisone injection might relieve pain in the joint for up to six months at a time.

STEP 6: LOOSEN UP BEFORE LOVEMAKING

If exercise takes some of the stiffness out of your joints, do some loosening up before lovemaking. You and your partner might want to exercise or stretch together.

STEP 7: MOIST HEAT HELPS

Take a warm shower or bath together before lovemaking, or try a bubble bath. Moist heat will help to loosen up your joints and diminish pain, and it can be a sensual experience as well.

If you enjoy applying body lotion to each other after your bath, this too can be a delightful prelude to lovemaking. A gentle body massage can also help you to feel more comfortable and more sensual.

STEP 8: YOU MAY NEED A
SEXUAL LUBRICANT

Some forms of arthritis can be accompanied by a condition called Sjögren's syndrome, which causes a decrease in secretions throughout your body, including vaginal lubrication. The lack of vaginal lubrication is part of your medical condition. It doesn't mean that you're not responding sexually.

If you should experience a decrease in vaginal lubrication due to your arthritis, a lovemaking oil or other sexual lubricant can make lovemaking much more comfortable. A commercially available lubricant that many of our patients like is Astroglide. Your pharmacist will probably carry it or will be able to order it. There are other preparations available as well. In an emergency a simple vegetable oil will work very well but will, of course, be more oily.

STEP 9: TAKE ADVANTAGE OF
COMFORTABLE POSITIONS

One of the ways that you can adapt your lovemaking to get around the problems of arthritis is to choose comfortable positions for intercourse. These will vary according to your specific needs.

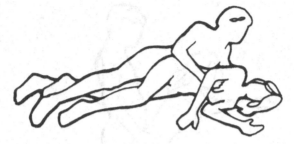

Figure 15-1. This illustrates what I'll call the "spoon position." Both partners lie on their sides with the man behind the woman. The man's penis enters the woman's vagina from behind. If it aids in comfort, the woman can place a pillow between her legs. Courtesy of the Arthritis Foundation

The standard "missionary position," in which the man supports himself over the woman while she lies with her legs spread, can be uncomfortable for a man if he has arm or shoulder problems, and it may be painful or even impossible for a woman with arthritis in her hips.

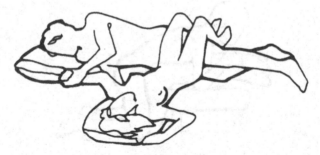

Figure 15-2. Here the woman lies on her back with her knees bent over her partner's hips. It's another helpful position if the woman has back trouble or difficulty spreading her hips or legs. It allows the partners to see each other and for the man to caress the woman's breasts during intercourse. Courtesy of the Arthritis Foundation

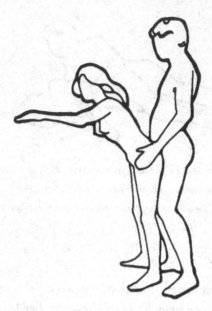

Figure 15-3. Both of you stand, with the woman leaning forward over a piece of furniture that is at a comfortable enough height for her to lean on for support and balance, while the man enters from behind. A pillow under her arms can provide extra comfort. Courtesy of the Arthritis Foundation

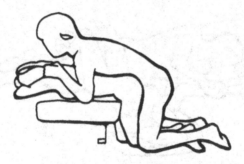

Figure 15-4. The woman kneels over a piece of low furniture, such as a soft hassock. Her knees may rest on a pillow for comfort. This position is helpful if she has hip problems, but it may be uncomfortable if her shoulders are affected. Courtesy of the Arthritis Foundation

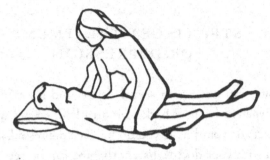

Figure 15-5. The man lies on his back while the woman kneels over him. He can use pillows to support his knees if desired. This is an especially good position if the man has hip, knee, or back complications. Courtesy of the Arthritis Foundation

The accompanying illustrations depict some positions that may be especially comfortable for people with arthritis. Look them over and choose the ones you can adapt to your own individual problems. (Actually, these positions might be worth a try whether or not you have arthritis.)

Pillows placed under your buttocks or knees will help in some positions. Knee pads, which can be purchased in most medical supply houses, can cushion painful joints.

The comfortable position in Figure 15-1 doesn't require either partner to support his or her weight on arms or knees. It's especially useful when the woman has hip involvement.

STEP 10: ORAL STIMULATION CAN SUBSTITUTE FOR ARTHRITIC HANDS

Arthritis in your hands may make difficult the kind of fine, gentle movements that you would like to use in caressing your partner. If this is the case, oral stimulation can be a very important substitute.

STEP 11: GET TREATMENT
FOR DEPRESSION

Depression can drain your sexual desire, and it's easy to get depressed when arthritis or back pain greatly interferes with important aspects of your life. If you do become depressed, discuss this problem with your doctor. Psychotherapy can be very important in helping you adjust to the changes in your life and self-image that can result from arthritis. Antidepressant medications can also help you to feel less depressed very rapidly—and this, of course, can help bring back your desire for lovemaking.

Remember, if one medicine doesn't work, don't give up! Another may, and there are new and better antidepressants being released all the time.

STEP 12: USE OTHER MEANS OF
STIMULATION WHEN YOUR ARTHRITIS
IS ESPECIALLY BAD

At times when arthritis flares up and becomes particularly troublesome you may find intercourse too uncomfortable, but you may still want to continue to enjoy mutual lovemaking for the intimacy it brings.

You and your partner can use manual or oral stimulation at these times to please each other sexually. Even when you don't feel well enough to enjoy being stimulated yourself, you may still wish to pleasure and satisfy your partner in this way. Consider the vibrator as another way to assist either of you to climax at times when intercourse is impossible (see chapter 12 for more information on vibrators).

STEP 13: MAINTAIN A POSITIVE
ATTITUDE TOWARD LOVEMAKING

In many cases it's not the physical problems that impair lovemaking as much as emotionally giving up. A strong desire to continue lovemaking can help you find a way around almost any physical impairment.

Don't feel locked into the positions for intercourse that you used before you developed arthritis or back trouble. Work on getting rid of preconceptions and prejudices about alternative ways of caressing, such as oral lovemaking. You may have to modify your lovemaking and use different methods of stimulation than you did before. Discard the inappropriate guilt feelings that you may have about making these changes in your lovemaking pattern. Some positive changes can result from your adversity; your lovemaking may end up more interesting and varied than before.

You may also feel guilty at times, because in having to abstain from intercourse you may fear you're also depriving your partner. If this happens, it's important that the two of you talk about it. Remember that you can satisfy your partner by other means, even if you're temporarily unable to have intercourse.

These thirteen steps won't make your physical difficulties disappear, but they can help you to keep your sexual life active and enjoyable, allowing you to continue to feel loved and loving—which is extremely important to each and every one of us.

CHAPTER 16

PAINFUL INTERCOURSE: IT'S NOT "ALL IN YOUR HEAD"

Most women experience occasional episodes of love-making in which intercourse is uncomfortable. Sometimes the discomfort subsides quickly, after the first few strokes. At other times, a slight discomfort may last throughout intercourse. This may not even be a problem for you if it doesn't interfere with your enjoyment.

But for some older women, the experience of chronic pain or discomfort during intercourse is a constant frustration. Their doctors often assume that their pain is caused by psychological factors if a physical cause isn't immediately obvious. And then even when a physical problem is found, they are likely to be told that their "mild" vaginal infection or "small" scar is insignificant and shouldn't be all that painful. The implication, then, is that since "nothing much" has been found, the problem is mostly mental.

On the contrary, just the opposite is usually true. The psychological problems that arise often result from the frustration of having real and chronic pain during sex, an activity that should be pleasant and enjoyable. Women who have pain with intercourse, a condition known as *dysparunia*, often *do* develop a negative attitude: "Sex just really hurts," blurted out a patient, after much evasion, "so why should I want it? There's no pleasure in it for me."

If you have repeated episodes of severe pain or discomfort with intercourse, you may develop a complication whereby the muscles around your vaginal opening go into involuntary spasm and clamp shut at the approach of your partner's penis. This is called *vaginismus*, and it can make intercourse impossible.

Vaginismus is an involuntary reflex. It's your body's way of flinching from pain. Sometimes vaginismus continues even when the original cause of the pain, such as an infection, is no longer present. Unfortunately, the vaginismus itself may then continue to make sexual attempts painful.

Although you may be having real pain, psychological factors can affect the way you perceive it. If, for example, you are generally unhappy about your relationship and you're not eager to make love, minor discomforts can become magnified, often without your realizing it.

Even when you are happy with your partner and desire lovemaking, anxiety about repeated pain can certainly create the beginnings of a vicious cycle: If sex has been consistently painful, you're bound to have apprehension about it, and that apprehension in turn can make you more sensitive to pain.

It may, then, be somewhat reassuring to hear that when a woman over forty who has enjoyed intercourse for years develops persistent severe pain on intercourse, there is probably a physical, treatable cause for it.

TYPES AND CAUSES OF PAINFUL INTERCOURSE

Painful intercourse, or dysparunia, is categorized into two types: *Superficial dysparunia* refers to pain felt at the opening of the vagina when the penis first penetrates. The pain may continue when the penis has fully entered. It's usually due to a vaginal problem or to vaginismus. On the other hand, *deep, or thrusting dysparunia*, does not usually involve any discomfort on initial entry but a great deal of pain when the penis thrusts against tender areas on the uterus, fallopian tubes, or surrounding structures deep inside the vagina.

Superficial Dysparunia   This condition is usually due to vaginitis or to lack of lubrication. In older women who are post-menopausal, it's usually caused by lack of estrogen, which produces atrophic vaginitis. This refers to thinning of the vaginal wall, with subsequent loss of the protective folds of the vaginal lining, loss of lubrication, and increased susceptibility to abrasion and infections. As described in our chapter on estrogen replacement therapy, atrophic vaginitis can usually be effectively treated by this means or by locally applied vaginal estrogen creams. If you can't use estrogens, vaginal lubricants may also be helpful.

Of course, other circumstances can account for insufficient lubrication in a woman of any age. They include lack of arousal, a feeling of being rushed, anxiety for any reason, or fear of recurrence of previous painful intercourse. Even the use of a tampon can cause a temporary dryness, because of its absorption of moisture.

Moreover, postmenopausal women, like women of any age, can develop a variety of common vaginal infections, which are another cause of superficial dysparunia. The most common are yeast infections (monilia) and trichomonal vaginitis. Some forms of vaginitis aren't apparent during routine gynecological exams, and so it may be necessary to take special vaginal smears, cultures, or other laboratory tests to find them. But once identified, they usually can be easily treated with antibiotics or other appropriate therapy.

Vaginitis can cause vaginal pain or burning, including burning on urination, and can continue for up to twenty-four hours after intercourse. This can certainly be enough to make a woman think twice about sexual relations, and even avoid them if it happens consistently.

Other infections that can cause pain include venereal warts, herpes lesions, and cysts or infections of the Bartholin glands. Venereal warts and herpes are usually sexually transmitted. Bartholin gland infections also may result from sexually transmitted infections.

A final cause of superficial dysparunia can be sensitive scars, whether from childbirth, episiotomy, or other prior surgery or traumatic injury.

Deep, or Thrusting, Dysparunia Pain with deep thrusting of the penis is often localized at a specific point or points of tenderness inside the vagina. It can sometimes be avoided by trying different positions for intercourse.

Endometriosis is a common cause of such pain in women who

are still menstruating. This condition, which results from growth of uterine tissue in the pelvic area outside the uterus, is never malignant. The uterine tissue responds to hormonal changes, which causes the pain to be most prominent when the woman is premenstrual.

Many women, even without endometriosis, find that around the time of their period their uterus is simply more tender and sensitive to deep thrusting during intercourse.

Other common causes for deep dysparunia in premenopausal women include pelvic infections, uterine myomas or cysts, and ovarian cysts or tumors.

Postmenopausal women are less likely to have many of these conditions, especially endometriosis, uterine myomas, ovarian cysts, or active pelvic infections. For them, atrophic vaginitis will be a more likely cause of deep as well as superficial pain, especially if they have not had estrogen replacement, since shortening of the vagina may make vigorous thrusting uncomfortable. Other causes of deep pain for older women include tumors of the uterus or ovaries and scarring or adhesions from old operations or from chronic pelvic infections.

Sometimes scars that are very tender are quite small in size. They may be passed over or felt to be insignificant during a routine gynecological exam, but they may be quite painful during intercourse.

Pelvic Congestion Syndrome This syndrome, another possible cause of dysparunia, is somewhat amorphous, controversial, and difficult to define. You may have an aching and a heavy feeling in your pelvis, but your gynecologist may not be able to find anything wrong. You may find thrusting during intercourse very painful.

Women with this syndrome often turn out to have either varicose veins in their pelvis, swelling in the broad ligaments of the uterus, scars and stretching from childbearing, or possibly a retroflexed uterus. The uterus appears normal, but these women seem to lose the pain after hysterectomy.

TREATMENT FOR DYSPARUNIA

The good news about both superficial and deep pain with intercourse is that there usually is something physical causing it, and there's often something that can easily be done about it.

First let's consider vaginismus. This, you remember, is a spasm of the muscles around the opening of the vagina as a protective involuntary reflex, due to a previous cause for painful intercourse. If that previous cause, such as a vaginal infection, is no longer present, excellent therapeutic results can be obtained with simple sexual therapy, using fingers or graduated vaginal probes to overcome the reflex.

If either deep or superficial dysparunia is due to atrophic vaginitis, the treatment is estrogen replacement. It can be fairly rapidly and spectacularly effective. Most forms of infectious vaginitis, on the other hand, are treated with antibiotics.

Endometriosis may be treated either medically or surgically. Medically it is treated hormonally with Danazol (danocrine), an androgen derivative that suppresses estrogen and causes the endometriosis patches to shrink and dry up; with Lupron, an analogue of gonadotropin-releasing hormone, which suppresses the pituitary's message to the ovaries and thus accomplishes the same estrogen suppression; or with other hormonal treatments involving high-dose birth control pills or progesterone. Various types of surgical treatments remove the endometriosis directly. Among these is a laser procedure that your gynecologist can best describe to you. Pelvic scars and adhesions are also usually treated surgically.

Keep in mind that while most of these conditions are treatable, they are often difficult to diagnose and therefore frustrating to deal with. It will take an understanding, intelligent doctor, as well as patience on both your parts, to help overcome them.

CHAPTER 17

SEX IN SPITE OF HEART TROUBLE: CONTINUE TO ENJOY IT

A simple and unpleasant fact of life is that, as we get older, we are more likely to suffer a heart attack or have to undergo a coronary bypass operation or other cardiac procedure, such as an angioplasty.

Men have many more heart problems than do women, and even a small one can have a traumatic effect on your sex life. A major cardiac problem such as a heart attack can cause you to lose your self-confidence and feel suddenly aged and afraid of exerting yourself. If this occurs, you may limit your sexual activity or develop impotence due to fear of causing another attack, due to angina or shortness of breath during sex, due to fatigue, or due to the side effects of medication.

A quarter of all men who have heart attacks give up sexual relations completely. Another 50 percent decrease the frequency of their sexual relations. Only the remaining quarter continue making love as often as before.

This is really a shame. It's not necessary or desirable to give up your sexual life after a heart attack. Resuming sex is good for your confidence, for your feeling of masculinity, for your sense of being a successful person, and for your entire outlook on life. Eighty percent of postcoronary patients can resume their normal sexual activity without any serious risks. The other 20 percent don't have to abstain from sex, but simply need to adjust their lovemaking style according to their exercise tolerance.

If you have had a heart attack or bypass operation, you may worry, "Will sex be too strenuous for me?" "Will my pulse rate go up too much?" "Will I get chest pain?" "Is sex safe for me?" You may even worry about dying during intercourse. You may well wonder, "Will lovemaking ever be the same again?"

The actual facts are reassuring. When a celebrity with a heart condition dies during sex with someone who is not his wife, it tends to make the scandal sheets. This may make it seem as if sex is something to worry about. Dying during sexual relations, however, is actually a rare occurrence. In a study of a large group of men with heart conditions who had died suddenly, *fewer than half of 1 percent* of them died during sex. Many more died in their sleep.

Moreover, of those few who did die during sexual relations, most were having sex with someone other than their usual partner and had also consumed large amounts of alcohol. The added stress in this kind of sexual situation can increase heart rate and blood pressure to much higher than usual levels, placing an extra burden on the heart.

HOW MUCH ENERGY CAN YOUR
BODY SAFELY EXPEND?

Medical research has developed fairly sophisticated methods of measuring what your body can do and how much energy it can expend safely. Energy expenditure is measured in metabolic units called METS. For example, washing your hands uses about two METS, while doing carpentry work uses five to six METS. Champion athletes can get their performance up to about twenty METS.

If you are an average middle-aged man who's had an uncomplicated myocardial infarction, you can probably exert eight to nine METS without developing chest symptoms. Sexual activity requires a lot less than that.

If you're having sex with your usual partner, you're likely to use about five METS during climax and about three to four METS during sexual play before and after climax. The energy level required for lovemaking is thus probably well within your capabilities.

Of course, sex varies in the amount of energy expended according to the intensity and excitement of the situation, but if you can, say, walk up two flights of stairs or their equivalent, you are doing about five to six METS, and you can most likely handle the physical requirements of sexual relations without much concern.

SEX DOESN'T NECESSARILY PRODUCE
YOUR PEAK PULSE RATE

Research on pulse rates during different activities has shown that ordinary daily activities often generate higher pulse rates than do sexual relations. In one study at Case Western Reserve School of

Medicine, men wore portable cardiac monitors throughout the day to record their pulse rate continuously. During the course of an ordinary day, these men developed a maximum pulse rate of 120 on average. By contrast, the highest pulse rate they had during sexual relations averaged only about 117. Even this rate only lasted around ten to fifteen seconds—during orgasm.

One forty-eight-year-old attorney, for example, demonstrated higher pulse rates walking to court, arguing with another attorney, and presenting a case in the courtroom than he did during sexual relations. We don't usually think of practicing law as a physically strenuous occupation, but an ordinary lawyer may put less strain on his heart making love than he does when engaged in his profession.

DISCOVER YOUR OWN
EXERCISE TOLERANCE

Knowing that lovemaking will probably be a low risk for you will help you return to enjoying it as much as you did before your heart condition. Here are some steps you can take to reassure yourself:

Check with Your Physician!   Make sure that you get adequate counseling from your physician about which activities you can tolerate and which ones you can't. It's important to get your questions answered. Worry can create tension during lovemaking that may hamper enjoyment and may even cause you to have difficulty functioning.

Have your partner present if possible, so her questions can be answered too. She may be apprehensive about causing you harm or pain, and her anxiety may inhibit her response, not to mention yours.

Some doctors ignore the issue of sexual activity after a heart attack. Even in today's world it's often because these doctors feel uncomfortable talking about sex, and sometimes it's because they have the misguided feeling that "at your age you shouldn't be worrying about sex."

If your doctor seems uncomfortable with the subject or doesn't seem to see it as a valid concern, ask to talk to another physician.

Know Your Limits   Lovemaking is a physical activity, a form of exercise like any other. So learn what your exercise tolerance is. With the help of a treadmill, as well as other tests, your doctor can evaluate you while checking your pulse rate and watching for arrhythmias. If you learn that you can tolerate a pulse rate of 140, for instance, and can climb several flights of stairs without getting anginal pain, then you probably can easily tolerate the exertion of sexual relations.

Get Yourself in Shape   Physical conditioning helps. Many cardiac rehabilitation programs offer physical conditioning designed specifically for men recovering from myocardial infarctions. Getting in better condition not only will make you feel physically stronger and more fit; it will also mean that your heart won't have to work as hard during sex.

HOW TO GO ABOUT RESUMING
SEXUAL RELATIONS

You will probably be advised to wait two to six weeks after your heart attack before resuming sexual relations. As much as you may be looking forward to lovemaking, the prospect may worry you too. These suggestions may make the transition easier:

Start Out Slowly   Alleviate some of your anxiety by taking a week for sexual caressing and petting without attempting intercourse. In this way, you and your partner can begin to enjoy lovemaking again without worrying about performance or pain. Climaxing from manual or oral stimulation usually takes less exertion and causes less increase in your heart rate and blood pressure than orgasm during intercourse does.

Be Comfortable and Relaxed   Resume sex in comfortable, familiar surroundings. Avoid trying sexual relations when you're under high stress or anxiety from your job or personal life. At these times your blood pressure and pulse rate may be higher to begin with, bringing with them higher risk.

Use Less Taxing Positions   Experiment with your partner to find less taxing positions for intercourse, such as one in which your partner is on top or in which the two of you are side to side. A comfortable alternative requiring minimal physical exertion is the spoon position, in which your partner lies on her side with her back toward you and you lie on your side behind her and insert your penis into her vagina from behind.

Lovemaking positions in which the man is on top, supporting his weight on his arms, do seem to require more energy than others. Remember, though, that the amount of energy used during lovemaking seems to be safe in most cases, no matter what position you use. So if you are partial to the "man-on-top" position and don't experience discomfort, there's probably no real reason for you to change.

Remember, intercourse isn't required for you to enjoy lovemaking. If you feel tired or unenergetic, use oral or manual petting to pleasure your partner or bring her to climax, and she can do the same for you.

CAN I TAKE VIAGRA?

If you don't have angina and have a healed myocardial infarction or cardiac bypass, there is probably no reason why you can't take Viagra. The question will be whether or not you can deal with the *physical exertion* of sexual relations, which we have discussed above. If you can handle the physical exertion, Viagra can help you resume sexual relations if you are having difficulty.

If you do have *angina* and require nitroglycerine or other nitrate medications, you *cannot* take Viagra.

On the other hand, if you are not taking nitrates and have taken Viagra, and should coincidently have some exacerbation of your heart problem, the doctors can work around the fact that you take Viagra as long as they know that you are on it. (A medical ID bracelet saying "I take Viagra" might be a worthwhile precaution.)

In all cases, if you have a heart condition, don't take Viagra without discussing it first, at length, with the doctor who is caring for your heart condition and knows the most about your status.

FOR WOMEN WITH HEART CONDITIONS

Although considerably less common, women do suffer heart attacks too. If this has happened to you, much of the same advice I've given to men will apply as well. Your ordinary daily activities probably cause levels of exertion as high as those you would experience during sex, but it would be important to find out what your actual exercise tolerance is through a treadmill test—and to ask your doctor specific questions about how you can enjoy sex without undue cardiac stress. A conditioning program would also probably be helpful for you.

Resume sex gradually, with just caressing at first, and start with positions that are less physically taxing for you until you can judge what will cause discomfort.

MEDICATIONS: SOME HELP, OTHERS MAY CAUSE PROBLEMS

Some medications that reduce painful heart symptoms can help you enjoy sex more. Others, also for your heart, can create sexual problems.

Some men *do* get anginal pain during sexual relations. In fact, this is one of the most common reasons that men give up sexual relations or develop impotence after a heart attack. If you do get angina during exertion, taking nitroglycerine or one of the longer-acting nitrates before making love may be helpful. Freeing your mind from the anticipation of pain will in turn make your lovemaking much more relaxed and enjoyable and will probably make it easier for you get erect.

It is very important to remember, though, that if you have angina during sex, and require nitroglycerine, you *cannot take Viagra.* It's the same if you take a longer-acting nitrate. Urologists tell me that some men on nitroglycerine, or other nitrates, lie to them about it in order to get Viagra. Don't do it! *This is a serious warning!* Taking Viagra with one of these medicines could kill you! (For more information about this serious medication interaction, review the information about erection and Viagra in chapters 1 and 2.)

Even if you need nitroglycerine for angina at other times but haven't needed it for sex, you almost certainly shouldn't take Viagra, because you never know when you might get angina and need your nitroglycerine. In any case, discuss it seriously with your cardiologist.

Although long-acting nitrates reduce your chances of getting angina, they also can cause sexual side effects for some people. If this happens, discuss possible alternatives with your doctor.

Beta blockers, such as Inderal, Tenormin, and Lopressor, cut down your maximum pulse rate during exertion and during intercourse and thereby decrease your chances of getting anginal pain. *Calcium channel blockers,* such as Adalat, Procardia, Isoptin, Calan, Cardizem, and others, can have the same effect. Unfortunately, these and some other medicines given to prevent arrhythmias can also have sexual side effects when taken in large doses, resulting in loss of sexual drive or ability to get erect. If this should happen to you, ask your doctor about substituting another medication. The recommended therapy will depend on your overall cardiac condition.

Many patients with heart problems have *high cholesterol* and are prescribed medicines to reduce their cholesterol levels. These medicines usually do not have any effect on erection or sexual desire. It is unlikely that you would have any sexual side effects from them.

Antihypertensives, for high blood pressure, are another class of medicines that are frequently prescribed for men with vascualar and heart trouble. Some of these, unfortunately, can cause sexual side effects. We will discuss these more in the next chapter and help you find the medicines that will be best for you.

OTHER RECOMMENDATIONS

Most physicians recommend that you don't have intercourse just after eating a large meal or consuming large amounts of alcohol. The considerable energy and blood flow being expended in digestion make less of both available for physical activity.

After a heart attack, many people become depressed and consumed with anxiety about their physical health. This loss of confidence and spirit can diminish sexual interest and desire. When you're worried and preoccupied, it's difficult to fully enjoy sex. If you are seriously depressed or anxious, an antidepressant or anti-anxiety medication may help you get back to functioning sexually as well as in the other spheres of your life.

Resuming sexual activity in any form can also actually help relieve some of your anxiety about your health. Sex is also an excellent reducer of anxiety in general and, whether you are a man or a woman, the feelings of closeness and intimacy achieved through satisfying lovemaking can impart a sense of well-being and fulfillment again.

If, after several months, you continue to feel depressed and unable to enjoy sex, it would be wise to ask your doctor to refer you to a psychiatrist who may be able to help you through this difficult period.

No one can guarantee that sex will be risk-free for you, and the risk can be higher at times of extra anxiety or excitement. It's a very small risk, though, taken for a very important reward. Every day you do many other things—like driving your car—that carry equal or greater risk. Life is meant to be lived, so if sex is important to you, go ahead and enjoy it and get the most out of it.

CHAPTER 18

CONTROLLING YOUR BLOOD PRESSURE WITHOUT LOSS OF SEXUAL FUNCTION

Some medications have side effects that commonly cause erection difficulties in older men. *Antihypertensives*, prescribed for high blood pressure, are among the most important and most commonly used medicines that cause sexual difficulty. Since they are so widely used, they are responsible for an inordinately high number of sexual problems, especially in older men. Literally hundreds of men over forty have come to me with erection difficulties due at least in part to antihypertensives.

It would be nice if patients could do without these medicines; however, those people who have high blood pressure *really need* antihypertensive medication, and really have no choice but to take it. Therefore it's easy to see why it is very important to know which blood pressure medicines are most likely to cause such problems and which ones are not. If this book can help you find the blood pressure medicines that cause the least trouble for you, it obviously will have done you a big service.

Unfortunately, one of my most challenging tasks in preparing this book was interpreting the research on hypertension and sexuality. The information on this subject is confused and contradictory. Every expert has a somewhat different opinion about which medicines are the worst offenders and which are the least. Not only that, blood pressure medicines are frequently changing, with new ones being introduced and old ones falling into disfavor. Definitive information on the incidence of sexual side effects from the newer medications is frequently unavailable. The good news is that some of the worst offenders among the older medications have now been replaced and are rarely, if ever, used.

What follows, then, is the result of my evaluation of the available studies, consolidated with my personal clinical experience and that of my consultants who work constantly with hypertensive patients.

THE FIVE MAIN CLASSES OF BLOOD PRESSURE MEDICATIONS

Different medications can cause different sexual problems. Some are more likely to cause failure of erection, some create difficulties with ejaculation, and others are responsible for loss of desire. Still others can provoke two or more of these problems. While the most visible sexual side effects, such as loss of erection, occur in men, it is not uncommon for women taking antihypertensive medications to suffer loss of sexual desire or difficulty with orgasm as well.

Many of the sexual side effects of antihypertensive medicines are dependent on the dose. If you can get away with a lower dose, you'll have a better chance of avoiding sexual side effects, so it's important to keep your weight down, to exercise, and to avoid salt.

As far as we know at the time of this writing, men who have erection difficulties from blood pressure medicines can safely take Viagra to help overcome these problems, as long as they are not also taking nitrates for angina. Again, check with your doctor. Viagra won't help with the lack of desire that can be caused by some blood pressure medicines. There are many more drugs in each class than I can list in this book, so if your blood pressure medication isn't listed below, ask your physician or pharmacist which class it belongs to. .

The Diuretics   Five main groups of high-blood-pressure medications are currently in fairly wide use. First are the *diuretics*—for example, Lasix (furosemide) and Dyazide (a combination of hydrochlorothiazide and triamterene). The diuretics are quite commonly used and are often among the first medicines tried in the treatment of high blood pressure. They generally work by increasing the secretion of salt and water in your urine.

The diuretics are generally felt to be fairly free of sexual side effects. They tend not to affect sexual desire and ejaculation, but the "thiazide" diuretics, such as hydrochlorothiazide, sometimes do cause erection problems.

The Sympathetic Blockers   The second group, the sympathetic blockers, is divided into several subtypes according to the mechanism of action.

The first subtype is the *beta blockers*, which include such medicines as Tenormin (atenolol), Lopressor (metoprolol), and Inderal (propranolol), as well as several others. "Beta" blocker refers to the type of nerve cell receptor that these medicines block to achieve their blood-pressure-lowering effect.

Beta blockers were once very commonly used, but they have now been largely replaced by newer medications.

The beta blockers tend to cause fairly frequent sexual side effects, including erection problems and loss of desire. However, as with all side effects, they don't affect everyone, and if one medication in this class causes trouble for you, it is still possible that another medication in the same class won't.

The *alpha blockers* include such medicines as Hytrin (terazosin) and Cardura (doxazosin). Interestingly, these two medicines have a dual usage. They are used both for the treatment of the symptoms of prostatic enlargement and for the treatment of hypertension. They work on hypertension by dilating the blood vessels and reducing vascular resistance. They tend not to cause any problems with erection but they can cause "retrograde ejaculation" in a few cases. If you have retrograde ejaculation, your ejaculated fluid goes backward into your bladder instead of coming out the end of your penis. This causes no harm, and the ejaculation *feels* pretty much the same as normal.

Minipress (prazosin) is another older alpha blocker which is now used much less frequently.

Trandate (labetalol) has both alpha- and beta-blocking effects. It does cause erection and desire problems at times, although perhaps somewhat less frequently than the pure beta blockers. *Other sympathetic blockers*, once widely used but now only rarely encountered, include Aldomet, Ismelin, and reserpine (Serpasil). These used to cause many more sexual side effects than the medicines now widely used.

Catapres (clonidine) is still used and can cause erection difficulties in up to 20 percent of men, loss of desire in both sexes, and inability to ejaculate in men and inability to climax in women.

The Calcium Channel Blockers This group of medications includes nifedipine (Procardia, Adalat), verapamil (Isoptin, Calan, Verelan), diltiazem (Cardizem, Dilacor), and half dozen more. (Some other trade names are Cardene, Nimotop, Plendil, Norvasc, and Dyna Circ.)

The calcium channel blockers have a number of uses, including treating high blood pressure, angina, and heart arrhythmias. When they were first introduced it was hoped that they would have far fewer sexual side effects than the beta blockers. Unfortunately, however, physicians who work with these medicines now feel that they also cause a fairly high incidence of erection difficulties.

The ACE Inhibitors The angiotensin-converting enzyme inhibitors (ACE inhibitors) are a newer class of medications that seem to be very well tolerated by most people. They seem to have few sexual side effects and therefore would be one of the best bets to start off with.

This class of drugs includes the following brand names: Accupril, Altace, Capoten, Lotensin, Monopril, Prinivil, Univasc, Vasotec, and Zestril. There are other brand names that are combinations of an ACE inhibitor and a diuretic or a calcium channel blocker.

The Angiotension II Inhibitors This class of medications, recently introduced, seems to have even fewer side effects, of all kinds, than the ACE inhibitors. It is rapidly becoming one of the most popular class of antihypertensives.

This group of medicines includes the following brand names: Cozaar, Diovan, Avapro, and others.

BEST BETS FOR CONTROLLING BLOOD PRESSURE WITH MINIMAL SIDE EFFECTS

No formula for treating blood pressure is right for everyone. The choices are now too wide, and they must be individualized for every patient. Nonetheless, I can try to present a rational course of action that can serve as a guideline for a man who wishes to control his blood pressure while conserving his sexual function.

1. *Weight loss, salt restriction, and exercise* may be enough to control your blood pressure without medication. At any rate, these are steps you can take yourself that will help you to minimize the amount of medication you will need.

2. *Quitting smoking and cutting down alcohol consumption* can have a marked effect on hypertension. Smoking immediately raises blood pressure and long-term smoking complicates arterial problems, while a heavy drinker with hypertension who quits drinking can see a drop in blood pressure of as much as fifteen points.

3. If you require medication, *an angiotensin II inhibitor, an ACE inhibitor, or a nonthiazide diuretic* would be a good place to start. Any one of these might control your blood pressure by itself with relatively few side effects, especially sexual side effects.

4. If the hypertension is still not controlled, you might have to add a beta blocker or calcium channel blocker. Remember that while these medications do cause sexual side effects for a substantial number of patients, there are plenty of patients for whom

they don't cause problems. And even if one beta blocker or calcium channel blocker causes sexual difficulty, another may not.

DON'T BE FRIGHTENED AWAY FROM ANTIHYPERTENSIVE MEDICATIONS

Hypertension is a major health problem and causes a greatly increased incidence of heart attacks, strokes, and kidney disease. But because it's a silent disease, people don't feel ill while the disease is progressing—until it reaches a very serious state. Because patients don't feel sick in the early and middle stages of hypertensive illness, they tend to be impatient with the side effects of the medications that treat it.

It's important for you *not* to be frightened off by the sexual side effects of antihypertensive medications. The frequency of such side effects is low with most of them and not universal with any of those routinely used today. Remember that a 5 percent incidence of sexual problems with a particular medicine means that 95 percent of the people taking it *don't* have sexual problems. Moreover, drug-related side effects, if they do occur, are reversible within a week or two after discontinuing the medicine.

We also know that a combination of different medicines and different classes of medicine allow for a lower dose of each and probably result in fewer overall side effects.

Even if one particular medicine does cause sexual side effects, another one may not. Frequently a change to another medication, even one from the same group, can overcome the problem. If your doctor is too rigid to do this or doesn't seem to care about your sexual difficulties, try another doctor.

Don't automatically assume that the blood pressure medicine you're taking is causing whatever sexual difficulty you may be having. Other very common causes of sexual difficulty that need to be evaluated include anxiety, stress, alcohol, smoking, diabetes, arteriosclerosis, other illnesses, and other medications.

Although I suggest various medications in this chapter, remember that your personal physician knows your case best and is best equipped to determine which medicines have the best chance of working for you, in the safest possible combinations.

CHAPTER 19

PRESCRIPTION MEDICINES
THAT CAN BLOCK
SEXUAL RESPONSE

As we reach the years over forty, we tend to be more vulnerable to sexual side effects from medications in general. This is partly because as we get older we have to take more medicines, and partly because at this age our sexual responses, especially those of males, become more fragile and more easily thrown off course by medication side effects.

Although some medications can cause women to have decreased sexual desire and impaired response, this condition is certainly less common than for men. This may be a result partly because women are less verbal about reporting sexual side effects, and partly because sexual impairment in women is harder to measure than a penis that doesn't rise. Unquestionably, however, a major part of the sexual disparity is due to the fact that women's sexual responses are not affected as much by aging as men's are.

This means that older men, with erection ability already a bit compromised, are simply more likely to be pushed past the threshold by a medication side effect.

Sexual function is a very complex process, and almost any drug that affects bodily processes can affect it on occasion. Trying to list every medication that could occasionally cause sexual side effects would be meaningless. And besides, new medications appear in every class all the time. What I hope will be more useful will be to briefly run through those *classes* of drugs in which sexual side effects are *most likely* to be seen.

THE ANTIHYPERTENSIVES

As we saw in the previous chapter, medications to control high blood pressure have been notorious in causing sexual problems. There are new classes of antihypertensives that seem much less troublesome, though. The problem of high blood pressure medicines is so important that if you are taking medications for high blood pressure, I'd advise that you read chapter 18 again carefully and discuss your options with your physician.

THE ANTIDEPRESSANTS

The Selective Serotonin Reuptake Inhibitors (SSRIs) are by far the most widely used class of antidepressants at present. These include such popular brand names as Prozac, Zoloft, Paxil, Celexa, and other related medications such as Effexor and Remeron.

These medicines tend to cause delay of ejaculation for some patients and even can cause complete blockage of ejaculation. In the same way, they can cause difficulty in achieving orgasm for women. Less frequently, these medications can cause erection problems. With longer-term use these medications can cause occasional loss of desire for patients of both sexes.

Tricyclic antidepressants and related compounds were once the most commonly used medications in the treatment of depression. They've been largely replaced by newer medications with fewer side effects. They are now used less frequently, mostly as adjuncts to the newer SSRI class.

Some of the widely known brand names of tricyclics include Elavil, Endep, Tofranil, Norpramin, Pamelor, Vivactil, Surmontil, Sinequan, and Ludiomil (generics: amitriptyline, imipramine, desipramine, nortriptyline, protriptyline, trimipramine, doxepin, and maprotiline).

These medications can cause sedation and decreased sexual desire in both men and women, as well as impotence in men in some cases. Impaired ejaculation has been reported, but it is less frequent.

The *monoamine oxidase (MAO) inhibitors*, another class of antidepressants, are now infrequently used because they can have more severe side effects. Two of the more commonly used MAO inhibitors are Nardil and Parnate (phenelzine and tranylcypromine).

The MAO inhibitors are less likely to affect sexual desire and erection, but they seem to cause impaired ejaculation fairly frequently. Inability to reach orgasm in women has also been reported.

The *miscellaneous antidepressants,* Desyrel, Serzone, and Wellbutrin (trazodone, nefazodone, and bupropion), are believed to have few or no sexual side effects. Desyrel, in fact, may improve erections, and there are some reports of Wellbutrin having similar effects.

Assessments of the sexual side effects of antidepressants are complicated by the fact that depression itself frequently causes lack of sexual desire or impotence. In fact, depression causes these symptoms considerably more frequently than do antidepressant medications. By treating the depression, the antidepressants actually help to restore sexual desire and sexual functioning in many instances.

For this reason, I certainly would not advise avoiding antidepressant medications because of the possibility of sexual side effects. If you need them, it's important to take them. And if one of them does cause sexual trouble, another may not.

OVER-THE-COUNTER COLD MEDICATIONS

Almost everyone has used *antihistamines* for treatment of colds, hay fever, allergies, or sinus trouble. These medications can be very useful, but their anticholinergic property that dries up your nose (which is the reason you take it) may also cause drying of vaginal secretions, and even impotence, though this is rather unlikely. Older men and women are particularly vulnerable to these side effects, though, as some postmenopausal women may already experience some decreased lubrication, and older men may have some erectile fragility.

Antihistamines are sometimes combined with *vasoconstricting medications* such as pseudoephedrine and others for the treatment of colds, and these vasoconstrictors can also be used separately, for example, Sudafed. Vasoconstrictors are also used in the nose drops that you may take to open your nose when you have a cold (phenylephrine and others).

These vasoconstricors can temporarily make it difficult to achieve an erection. You are using them for your nose, but they travel in your bloodstream all over your body. Their effect, to constrict blood vessels, works fine to open your nose, but it has the opposite effect on the vasodilation that you need in your penile blood vessels in order to get an erection. The effect is absolutely temporary, and your erection ability will return as soon as your cold is enough better so that you can stop the cold medications.

Thus, if you are taking a vasoconstrictor temporarily for a cold and you find that your penis just won't get erect, *don't be alarmed.* This is a natural side effect of the medication, and it will disappear when you stop the medication.

ULCER MEDICATIONS

Tagamet (cimetidine) is a medication that used to be very commonly prescribed for the treatment of ulcers and other forms of gastrointestinal distress. Unfortunately, it also has antisexual effects on men, because it blocks the effect of the androgens, or male hormones, causing sexual side effects.

The good news is that Tagamet has largely been replaced by Zantac (ranitidine) and Prilosec (omeprazole), which don't have antiandrogen effects. If Tagamet has caused sexual problems for you, you might ask your doctor about Zantac or Prilosec.

OTHER MISCELLANEOUS DRUGS

Major tranquilizers, sometimes called neuroleptics or antipsychotics, are prescribed primarily for serious psychiatric conditions, but they are occasionally given in low doses for other symptoms.

The older neuroleptics, such as Thorazine, Stelazine, Trilafon, Mellaril, and Haldol, can interfere with sexual desire and erection. They may also raise the levels of prolactin, a pituitary hormone, which suppresses male sexual hormones. Some can occasionally cause impaired ejaculation or orgasm. Again, older men and women can be more vulnerable to these side effects.

Fortunately, the newer neuroleptics, such as Zyprexa (olanzapine), seem to have far fewer sexual side effects and have largely replaced the older medications.

Common antianxiety medications, such as Xanax and Valium, may decrease sexual desire, especially when taken in high doses.

Other medications that occasionally cause sexual difficulty include muscle relaxants, medications for Parkinson's dsisease, and such miscellaneous medicines as Lanoxin, Dilantin, Reglan, Flagyl, Indocin, and Atromid-S. The reason that some of these medicines affect sexual response is obscure.

Sexual side effects for men can be either an inability to achieve erection or a loss of desire. Again, as I wrote in the previous chapter, as far as we now know, Viagra can be used safely in combination with other medications (except nitrates and nitroglycerine) to help overcome problems of erection ability, but it will not be able to improve loss of desire.

IN SUMMARY

As I explained at the beginning of this chapter, I have not tried to list all medications that could possibly cause trouble. What is important for you to remember is that if you start having sexual problems, go over your medications with your doctor, especially if you have recently started a new medication in one of the categories that I have mentioned, and see if you can substitute one with fewer sexual side effects.

Again, remember that just because you're taking one of the medicines listed here doesn't mean you are likely to have sexual difficulties. And if you are taking one of these medicines and do have sexual difficulties, there's no assurance that the medicine is necessarily responsible for the problem, unless it clearly started shortly after you began taking the drug.

Finally, remember that medication side effects are almost always completely reversible simply by discontinuing the medication and substituting another one.

CHAPTER 20

DRINKING, SMOKING, DRUGS, AND SEX OVER FORTY

You may get the feeling that there is a constant barrage of voices telling you that some of your favorite things, such as alcohol and smoking, are bad for you. Much as I regret adding my voice to the others, I must. If you drink or smoke heavily, this chapter will not be what you want to hear. In fact it may be quite upsetting. But unpleasant as this information is, it's crucial for you to hear it, if you want to maintain a good, active sexual life.

WHAT ARE THE LONG-TERM SEXUAL EFFECTS OF ALCOHOL CONSUMPTION?

At some time or other, you've probably had a drink or two before a lovemaking episode and felt that it helped you to relax and to be more uninhibited. But what about the effects of three or four drinks, or more, on your sexual ability when you're over forty? And what are the effects of heavy or chronic alcohol use?

I wish that I could tell you that alcohol is perfectly safe and won't cause you any sexual trouble. Unfortunately, that's simply not the way it is. All the medical evidence indicates that alcohol, in large amounts, can be extremely destructive to your sexual life. A pint of hard liquor per day, or an equivalent amount of alcohol as wine or beer, can cause complete loss of sexual function in as few as five to eight years. As many as 80 percent of men who drink very heavily are reported to develop impotence, sterility, or loss of sexual desire.

Heavy drinking seems to be especially toxic to the male sex glands, the testicles. Over a long period of time, it destroys the cells and leaves you with atrophic (shrunken) testicles. One of your testicles' main functions is to produce the male hormone testosterone. As we described in an earlier chapter, testosterone regulates sexual desire and potency. Overuse of alcohol for a long period of time can greatly decrease production of testosterone. This may result in loss of sexual desire and even impotence.

The testicles also produce sperm. As excessive alcohol consumption gradually destroys your testicles, it causes you to have a lowered sperm count, which will eventually make you sterile and thus unable to father a child. This may still be an important consideration for many over-forty men.

HOW ALCOHOL LOWERS YOUR MALE HORMONE LEVELS

Alcohol actually decreases your working levels of testesterone in three ways.

First of all, it decreases the production of testosterone in your testicles, as just described.

Second, it alters your metabolism by increasing the rate at which testosterone is broken down in your body. In doing so, it changes your body's hormone balance. Men who drink very heavily have less male hormone and more female hormone than normal. (Men normally have small amounts of female hormones in their bodies, just as women have small amounts of male hormones.)

Third, alcohol increases the percentage of testesterone in your blood that's tightly bound to protein. This means that less of it is free and able to act. Thus, not only is there a reduced amount of testosterone produced, but part of what is produced isn't usable.

Besides its effects on the testicles, alcohol damages your liver, and this damage helps to produce the hormonal imbalance with excess female hormones. Alcohol may also have toxic effects on the areas of the brain that help regulate sex hormones, disrupting the production of the pituitary hormones that stimulate the testicles to produce testosterone and sperm.

Remembering that testosterone levels usually decrease with age anyway—and that your liver gradually loses some of its efficiency even without alcohol—you can see how heavy drinking after forty can be even more debilitating than when you were younger.

IS THE DAMAGE PERMANENT?
WILL IT HELP IF I STOP DRINKING?

Two types of damage result from chronic alcohol abuse. The first is the change in your body's biochemistry, which causes you to have lowered levels of male hormone. This change can be reversed if you stop drinking, although it will take some time.

The second is the permanent destruction of the cells of the testicles and liver. This probably takes heavy drinking over a long period of time, but once it occurs, it's not reversible. Once cells are killed and scarring takes place, that's it.

So while many men can regain sexual function within several months if they quit drinking, for others it may be too late. It seems to depend on the amount of cell damage in the testicles and liver that has already occurred. Men with atrophic testicles and damaged livers are unlikely to have a return of sexual function from just stopping drinking. But the earlier you stop heavy drinking, the better your chances. Even if you don't get a full return of function, at least you will prevent further damage.

EVEN ONE EPISODE OF EXCESSIVE DRINKING CAN AFFECT YOU

The negative results of alcohol on sexuality don't affect only those who happen to be alcoholics. Early signs of damage can be seen after a single episode of excessive drinking. Enough alcohol to produce a hangover can cause temporarily decreased testosterone levels even in normal, healthy men.

Alcohol has other immediate effects. It serves as a depressant to the central nervous system, and as such in small doses it decreases your inhibitions and allows you to relax. But in higher doses, it deadens your nervous system. This means that you become less sensitive and more sedated. Alcohol thus numbs the reflex pathways that your body depends on for sexual response. It ends up causing sexual failure.

This deadening effect of high doses of alcohol on sexuality has been well proven. For example, the more alcohol that men have consumed in the previous twenty-four hours, the more their nighttime erections decrease in size and frequency, and the more alcohol they consume before watching sex films, the fewer and smaller erections they're measured to have. This is the opposite of what men often expect, which is that alcohol will help them to get erect.

The immediate sexual-suppressing effect from a single dose of alcohol can cause a man lasting sexual difficulties. For example, after a party at which he had consumed a particularly large amount of alcohol, Bill W., a patient of mine, came home and attempted to have sex with his wife. Unfortunately, due to the alcohol, he completely failed to get an erection.

The next morning he remembered what had happened, and he worried for the next two days about his failure. When he tried again, his worry caused another failure and more worry. His single episode of alcohol-created impotence snowballed into the prolonged period of sexual difficulty that eventually brought him to my office.

This pattern of alcohol-induced failure, leading to anxiety about performance and more failures, is not at all uncommon, and it can affect women as well. After heavy alcohol consumption causes failure of arousal or orgasm, a woman may consciously watch her response and try harder to get aroused the next time. This usually has the opposite effect and can get her into the same vicious circle of anxiety and sexual difficulty that Bill W. suffered.

MEN OVER FORTY ARE
PARTICULARLY VULNERABLE

Older men are especially susceptible to the detrimental effects of alcohol on potency. As you age, your erection reflex gets more fragile, and an amount of alcohol that would have caused no problem in earlier years may be enough to tip the balance to loss of function. When you were younger, your erection reflex was so strong that you could get erect under almost any circumstances, in spite of the deadening effects of alcohol. Now you simply don't have the reserve that you once had. Your testosterone levels have declined with age, and neither the vascular supply to your penis nor the nerve stimulation is as strong as it used to be. You can't afford to have your testosterone levels further lowered by alcohol. You also can't afford to deaden your senses with alcohol and expect to function well. You need to give yourself all the advantage you can, instead of letting alcohol make it difficult or impossible for you to get erect.

AND WOMEN?

The effects of alcohol on women in many ways parallel those on men. Immediately, a small amount of alcohol, such as one or two drinks, may relax your inhibitions, which may allow you to feel more sexually aroused. However, after three to five drinks you may have considerable difficulty in climaxing because of the deadening effects of alcohol on your nervous system. With much more alcohol, you will likely become quite intoxicated, fall asleep, or even pass out.

Chronic alcohol abuse is toxic to the ovaries, the female sexual glands, in the same way that it's toxic to the testicles. Damage to the ovaries causes menstrual abnormalities, lack of ovulation, and signs of estrogen deprivation. The lack of estrogen can cause atrophy of the breasts, uterus, and vaginal walls, along with loss of lubrication. Alcoholic women also suffer from chronic liver disease, premature aging, and early menopause. Masters and Johnson report that 30 to 60 percent of alcoholic women claim difficulty in becoming sexually aroused, impaired orgasm, and other sexual problems.

DOES THIS MEAN I SHOULDN'T DRINK AT ALL?

You may be wondering, "What does this mean to me? Do I have to stop drinking completely? Will an occasional drink or two cause me any trouble? How long will it take for heavy drinking to cause problems for me sexually?"

It should be emphasized that most of the data referred to here involve studies done on chronic heavy drinkers. These are not skid-row alcoholics, though. I see people like them with sexual problems every day—"ordinary folks" who live with their families, go to work every day (or almost every day), but who "like to drink." If you are one of these people, this kind of damage could be happening to you.

There's considerable individual variation in susceptibility to damage from alcohol. Not everyone who drinks a pint a day for six or seven years will become impotent. On the other hand, some people may experience loss of function from much smaller amounts, or after drinking for a shorter time.

While there is lots of evidence that a large amount of drinking, even on a single occasion, will cause a temporary drop in testosterone and a temporary inability to function sexually, there is no indication that one or two drinks a couple of times a week will cause any loss of sexual function.

What I'd advise, therefore, is very simple:

1. If you've had decreased sexual function and you've been drinking moderate to heavy amounts, try discontinuing for at least three or four months to see if your function returns.

2. If you've been drinking heavily and you haven't yet suffered a loss of function, you're in luck: You can cut down or quit now before it's too late.

3. If you're concerned about your sexual function, I suggest you limit yourself to a maximum of one or two drinks before a sexual encounter, and keep your total alcohol consumption light.

HOW SMOKING CIGARETTES CAN SUPPRESS YOUR SEXUAL FUNCTIONING

The effects of cigarette smoking on sexual functioning have not been as thoroughly studied as have the effects of alcohol. There is little known, for example, about the effect of smoking on female sexual response. There is, however, considerable evidence that smoking has damaging effects on a man's erection ability, both immediate and long term. In fact, a well-known impotence researcher once stated that *"smoking may be the most important risk factor for erection problems."* He noted that about 80 percent of the impotent men he treated were smokers. A large proportion of impotent men in my own practice are smokers as well. When you consider that smoking increases the risk of cardiovascular disease and hypertension, and that these both can be factors in causing impotence, it is not such a surprising observation.

Smoking *as few as two* high-nicotine cigarettes before sexual arousal can cause decreased erection as well as slower arousal, even in healthy young men. This effect is probably caused by the immediate vasoconstrictive effects of nicotine—meaning that nicotine constricts the small blood vessels in your penis, reducing the blood supply and thereby delaying or preventing erections.

There is also evidence that impotent men may be much more likely to be smokers than the general population, and the incidence of heavy smoking among impotent men is much greater than that in the general population. Heavy smokers also tend to have decreased blood pressure in their penises, confirming the impaired blood supply that contributes to impaired erections. The evidence shows that men who have smoked the longest and have smoked the most cigarettes per day have the lowest penile blood pressures.

Overall, this implies that cigarette smoking is clearly a risk factor in producing impotence as well as many other medical problems. The way it affects men seems to be largely vascular, by narrowing and obstructing the blood vessels needed to produce erection.

What if you quit smoking? A study several ago, which was published in the journal *Urology*, examined men who were impotent due to what the researchers felt were vascular causes. Some of them had diabetes. In others, there was no clear-cut cause for their impotence except for the fact that they smoked a pack and a half or more of cigarettes per day.

The investigators felt that there was good evidence that smoking caused constriction of the blood vessels and that it was contributing to the men's sexual problems. The men were asked to discontinue smoking for a trial period. It was found that 35 percent of these men with proven impotence had their problems reversed within six weeks—by simply not smoking for that period of time.

It's clear that stopping smoking won't reverse impotence in everyone. But it is striking that more than one-third of these men experienced a return of erections *with no other treatment* than stopping smoking.

So if you value your continued sexual function, keep in mind that there is considerable evidence that by smoking a pack or more of cigarettes per day you are endangering it. The longer you smoke and the more you smoke, the more you're probably endangering yourself. The sexual-suppressing effect probably occurs because nicotine constricts the blood vessels and smoking increases hardening of the arteries (arteriosclerosis). I'm well aware that smoking is a very difficult addiction to break and that quitting isn't easy, but endangering your sexual life by smoking isn't pleasant to contemplate either.

Certainly the relationship between drinking and smoking and sexuality is complex and interwoven with social factors and attitudes. Cutting down on drinking and quitting smoking won't guarantee that your sexual response will never be impaired, or that it will be restored if you are currently having trouble. It again comes down to the fact that, as you get older, it makes sense to maximize your chances for good sexual functioning by eliminating factors that can potentially cause major impairment—and alcohol abuse and smoking are definitely in that category.

STEROIDS FOR MUSCLE BUILDING

Some muscle builders and athletes take anabolic steroids related to testosterone to try to gain more muscle mass. Taking these hormones raises their levels in your bloodstream, of course. This fools the receptors in your brain into thinking that there is no further need for testosterone, and the brain stops putting out the hormone-messengers that tell your testicles to keep working. The testicles shut down, shrink, and atrophy. One of the urologists I work with told me of a nice young man in his early twenties who came in with shriveled testicles. In effect, the urologist told me, the young man had been effectively castrated by using these drugs. Just to be better in sports! Enough said.

"RECREATIONAL" DRUGS

The use of recreational drugs has become all too common in our society—even, in some cases, among men and women over forty. I would be remiss if I didn't mention some of the sexual effects—and dangers—of the most common of these drugs.

The short-term sexual effects of psychoactive drugs are extremely variable and depend a lot on the social setting. For the most part, however, the occasional use of small amounts of such drugs as marijuana, cocaine, and amphetamines may be experienced as reducing inhibitions and increasing sexual sensitivity. As with alcohol, though, the ingestion of larger amounts of these drugs tends to interfere with such sexual responses as erection, ejaculation, and female orgasm—while chronic, steady use tends to cause progressive loss of sexual desire for both sexes, resulting in inability to reach erection or ejaculation for men and inability to reach orgasm for women.

Heroin and other narcotic opiates are sexual suppressants in almost any dose.

Marijuana   Marijuana is commonly thought to have an aphrodisiaclike effect. About 80 percent of both men and women in a large study by Masters and Johnson reported that marijuana enhanced their enjoyment of sex. More specific questions, however, determined that what was enhanced was sensory perception and the feeling of relationship with one's partner. Actual sexual functions, such as erection ability, ejaculation, vaginal lubrication, or female orgasm, were not improved. In fact, they were actually interfered with in many cases, especially when high doses had been taken. As with alcohol, a small amount may have released inhibitions, but larger amounts tended to cause inability to get erect, ejaculate, or reach orgasm.

With chronic use, marijuana is an antisexual drug. In animals it decreases copulation activity, suppresses the production of sperm and testosterone in males, and prevents ovulation in females. In humans it definitely causes marked suppression of testosterone levels and decreases sperm counts. It can cause loss of sexual desire, inability to ejaculate and impotence in men who are chronic users, and loss of desire and inability to reach orgasm in women. In one study of daily users, one out of five was impotent.

Cocaine   Highly valued in the drug culture as a sexual stimulant, cocaine reduces inhibitions and apparently can increase sexual desire in both men and women in the short run. It also increases tactile sensation and can prolong intercourse by delaying ejaculation.

With chronic usage, however, there is first an inability for men to ejaculate or for women to reach climax, then loss of male erection ability and female arousal, and finally, after a few months, complete loss of sexual interest for both sexes. This is probably due to the drug's depletion of dopamine, a specific neurotransmitter in the nervous system.

The initial effects of cocaine can be seductive, but this is a very dangerous drug. A single dose can be fatal. Besides this, it is highly, highly addictive. I have seen people in my practice who thought they could just be social users but who became compulsively addicted, ruining their marriages, losing their jobs, and bankrupting themselves. *Beware of cocaine!*

Amphetamines (Speed)   Much less scientific data are available on the effects of amphetamines on sex. Like cocaine, however, these are central nervous system stimulants. Anecdotal reports indicate that amphetamines have many of the same initial effects as cocaine as well as similar long-term dangers and side effects.

Opiates and Narcotics (Heroin)   The sexual story on opiates is pretty clear-cut. Opiates will decrease sexual desire and function in almost 100 percent of regular users. Both men and women lose the ability to become aroused. Men develop impotence. Women can't climax. Testosterone and pituitary sex hormones are depressed in men. Women stop ovulating and develop amenorrhea. Opiates are definitely a sexual downer.

CHAPTER 21

PROSTATE PROBLEMS, SEX,
AND THE OLDER MAN

With aging, some prostate trouble is almost inevitable for most men. Unfortunately, though, when many men think of prostate trouble they think of frightening operations, loss of sexual function, and embarrassing urinary symptoms. You'll be glad to hear that it doesn't have to be that way at all. In fact, you can continue to have good sex indefinitely in spite of prostate trouble.

Prior to age forty, your prostate gland is likely to cause you little difficulty besides an occasional prostate infection. However, by your fifties or sixties, you will probably start noticing symptoms caused by enlargement of your prostate gland such as urgency and frequency of urination, difficulty in starting your urinary stream, and difficulty in turning it off completely so that you may have some dribbling after urinating.

WHAT IS THE PROSTATE GLAND?

Your prostate is a small gland located between your bladder and the base of your penis. It actually fits like a small doughnut around your urethra (the passage you urinate through) where your urethra leaves your bladder. This area is called the bladder neck. The rectum is right behind it, so your doctor can easily feel your prostate during a rectal exam.

The prostate is normally about one and a half to two inches in size, and it weighs about half an ounce. Severely enlarged prostates can be fifteen times this size and weigh as much as half a pound.

Only men have a prostate gland. It grows to its full size at puberty, under the stimulation of your male sex hormones, just like your other sex organs. It is composed, for the most part, of glandular tissue with a fibrous and muscular capsule.

Your prostate is constantly at work producing enzymes, hormonelike substances, and, most important, the alkaline fluid that comprises most of your ejaculation. This fluid helps the sperm to swim once they reach the vagina.

A small amount of this prostatic fluid is usually voided every time you urinate so it won't build up in your prostate. Your prostate produces more fluid than usual when you are sexually excited, to ensure an adequate supply for ejaculation. If you go for a long period of time with frequent episodes of excitement but no ejaculation, your prostate may become painfully congested with fluid. While not dangerous, this can be very uncomfortable.

PROSTATIC ENLARGEMENT, OR "BPH"

For reasons that nobody fully understands, most men's prostates begin to grow again at about the age of forty or fifty. This causes prostatic enlargement, also called benign prostatic hypertrophy or BPH. BPH represents the enlargement of the glandular, fibrous, and muscular tissue inside the capsule of your prostate. It doesn't spread into other tissue, it's not invasive, and it's not cancerous.

BPH really isn't any danger in itself, but your enlarged prostate may start to obstruct your urinary tract, which passes through it. In extreme cases, the obstruction may completely block your urine outflow. Since BPH starts very gradually and causes symptoms only if it obstructs your urine, you can have it for a long time and never even know it.

The symptoms caused by blockage due to BPH include some or all of the following: a need to urinate more often than usual during the night, difficulty in starting your urinary stream, slowness and weakness of your stream, a need to urinate frequently and with great urgency, painful or uncomfortable urination, dribbling of urine after urination, and passing small amounts of blood in your urine or ejaculate.

The good news is that BPH usually doesn't interfere with your sexual activity except perhaps for a slight decrease in the force of your ejaculation. When BPH is accompanied by congestion, in rare cases it may cause erection difficulty, but this is very unlikely.

Again, what causes BPH isn't clear. Male hormones have to be present for the prostate to enlarge, but they were present in much higher amounts when you were younger. Dietary factors may be related to BPH. Japanese men on a traditional fish diet with low cholesterol have a low incidence of BPH and of prostatic cancer. When they come to this country or switch to a diet high in saturated fats, the same men get more prostatic enlargement and more prostate cancer.

Some doctors believe that the body nutrient zinc may play a factor. Zinc is highly concentrated in the prostate and seems to play a role in its proper function. There is a hypothesis that the prostate enlarges in response to low zinc levels, the same way that the thyroid enlarges in response to low iodine levels, but there is really no good evidence for this. It is simply a theory with an appealing rationale, but no proof.

There is considerable evidence that older men can develop zinc deficiency, so some people deduce that taking supplementary zinc in doses of about 50 milligrams per day may help prevent prostate enlargement. As I stated above, it's very difficult to find any scientific studies proving this. Many men take zinc for their prostate because they and their doctors hope that it will be beneficial, but it's not a medically proven treatment at this time.

THE NEW ORAL TREATMENTS FOR BPH

When I wrote the first edition of this book twelve years ago, the standard, and pretty much the only, treatment for symptomatic BPH was surgery. Now most patients avoid surgery thanks to new *oral agents* that can relieve symptoms.

Many studies have shown that the severity of symptoms of BPH and the amount of urinary obstruction aren't simply related to the size of the enlarged prostate. There is another factor, an increase in tone of the smooth muscle in the prostate and the bladder neck, and this increased tightness of the muscle obstructs the urine as it leaves the bladder.

Hytrin (terazosin) and Cardura (doxazosin)   are alpha-I blockers, and their action relaxes the smooth muscle in the prostate and bladder neck, thus allowing the urine out and relieving the symptoms although there is no change in the prostate size. These medicines are dual purpose as they can both be used to treat high blood pressure as well. Sexual side effects seem to be minimal.

Flomax (tamsulosin) is a newer medicine of a related class, which only relaxes the prostate and bladder neck and doesn't drop blood pressure, thus avoiding some of the low-blood-pressure side effects that some men might experience with Hytrin or Cardura. Depending on the dose, up to 20 percent of patients report ejaculation disturbances. There are no reports of erection or libido problems.

Proscar (finasteride) is a medication that works on the size of the prostate instead of relaxing the smooth muscle. It inhibits the conversion of testosterone to 5-alpha dihydrotestosterone (DHT), which is a powerful androgen and seems to be a prime factor in causing prostatic enlargement. Proscar causes reduction in the size of the prostate and also causes symptom relief. It tends to be used primarily for men with very large prostate glands. Probably because of its effect on testosterone Proscar can cause impotence, loss of desire, and decreased amount of ejaculate for some patients.

Another very interesting treatment for the symptoms of benign prostatic enlargement is the use of herbal extracts from the *saw palmetto plant*. This is widely prescribed in Europe, although much less frequently here. It may work, at least partly, by the same mechanism as Proscar (finasteride), in inhibiting the conversion of testosterone to dihydrotestosterone.

In a large double-blind multicenter study comparing Proscar with saw palmetto extracts (*Serenoa repens*), the two treatments proved equally effective in the management of BPH. Symptom relief was equal. The patients treated with saw palmetto don't seem to have as much improvement in parameters such as flow rates, residual urine, reduction in prostate size, and PSA values, but they do *feel* as good with equal reduction in symptoms and feeling of improvement in the quality of life. The patients on saw palmetto also have a lower incidence of sexual side effects (impotence, loss of desire, blockage of ejaculation) than the patients on Proscar.

Saw palmetto extracts are available in health food stores, but this could result in a real danger for you. If you treat your prostate symptoms yourself, without regular urological evaluations, you could have a prostate *cancer* and not know it. Get your prostate exam!

SURGICAL TREATMENTS FOR BPH

Prostatic surgery may be needed in the treatment of BPH if the prostate enlargement is causing blockage of the urinary tract. The surgery may be an ordinary surgical procedure such as a transurethral resection (TUR), a suprapubic prostatectomy, or a retropubic prostatectomy, or it could be an endoscopic ablation using lasers, radio waves, or microwaves to remove tissue instead of using physical means.

We will start with a *TUR*, or *transurethral resection*, as that is still the gold standard for surgical treatment of BPH. In this procedure an instrument is inserted through your urinary passageway back to your prostate and bladder. Some of the enlarged prostate tissue is then cut away to widen the passage through which you urinate. This alleviates the blockage of urine and allows you to urinate more easily. It is the simplest operation and leaves no scar. It now usually requires just an overnight stay in the hospital and is preferred for most ordinary cases of prostatic hypertrophy.

For very enlarged prostates, either *a suprapubic prostatectomy* or *a retropubic prostatectomy* is performed. These operations are both called "open" prostatectomies because they involve abdominal incisions. The suprapubic operation involves approaching the prostate through the bladder, while the retropubic essentially goes under the bladder.

None of these operations is likely to cause interference with your erection ability. Most patients return to having intercourse three to six weeks after surgery. However, all of these procedures cause a condition known as *retrograde ejaculation*.

Let me explain what retrograde ejaculation is: When you ejaculate, your prostate ordinarily expels semen into your urethra. Your bladder-neck sphincter muscle closes so that the ejaculation can't flow backward into your bladder. The ejaculation is then forced out the end of your urethra.

Now all three of the operations we discussed open and widen your bladder neck surgically. This is done to remove the blockage that was causing those uncomfortable urinary symptoms and to allow the urine to pass, but it also affects your ejaculation: In most patients, the bladder neck remains permanently open and doesn't fully close during ejaculation. This means that almost all the ejaculation fluid will flow backward into the bladder, instead of being expelled from the penis.

This backward flow is called retrograde ejaculation, which means simply "ejaculation backward." It doesn't cause any harm, and the ejaculation fluid comes out later, during urination.

Retrograde ejaculation does not significantly decrease the sensation of orgasm, since it is the contractions of the prostate and the penis that give the sensation, and they aren't changed. It feels pretty much the same, and many men don't even realize that it's happened until sometime afterward, when they notice that no fluid was expelled.

Several oral medications, which are alpha adrenergic agonists (stimulants) and thus smooth-muscle constrictors, have recently been discovered to improve bladder-neck tone and allow the semen to be expelled from the penis during orgasm in some patients. The most common of these is phenylpropanolamine, but pseudoephedrine will also work. They are commonly used in cold tablets and, if taken regularly, could have side effects such as raising blood pressure, causing anxiety, and others. Ornade is a common over-the-counter cold medicine containing phenylpropanolamine but it also contains an antihistamine that causes drying and some sedation. Another medication that can work is the antidepressant imipramine.

If you are having retrograde ejaculation subsequent to a prostate operation, check with your physician to see if phenylpropanolamine or one of the other medications would be indicated for you. Don't be too surprised if your doctor is not initially familiar with this treatment for retrograde ejaculation, because it is not known by everybody.

ENDOSCOPIC TREATMENTS FOR BPH

These treatments are sometimes used as a substitute for a transurethral resection (TUR) operation. They involve inserting a small tube into the urethra and then, instead of surgically removing tissue, they use either a *laser*, or *radio waves* (trans-urethral needle ablation, or TUNA), or *microwaves* (trans-urethral microwave therapy or TUMT), to create heat and burn away tissue.

All these treatments require less anesthesia than a TUR and can often be done on an outpatient surgery basis. Unfortunately, the endoscopic treatments may require reoperation because they don't take as much tissue as the TUR, and therefore symptoms may come back.

PROSTATE INFECTION

Prostate infection, called *prostatitis*, is a common illness in men, and it may occur at any age.

Acute Bacterial Prostatitis usually strikes with the sudden onset of fever, chills, nausea, vomiting, inability to start urinating, or painful, burning urination. You may feel as if you have to urinate with great urgency and frequency, but you may produce only small amounts of urine. You may also have rectal pain and low-back pain. Because it can be quite serious, it's important to consult with your doctor as soon as possible after the onset of symptoms.

Once an infection gets into the prostate, it's difficult to completely eliminate it. The prostate doesn't empty well. It's hard for antibiotics to get into this area, and it's hard for prostatic fluid to get out. Little pockets of infection remain resistant to treatment.

Chronic Recurring Prostatitis, which may or may not start with an acute infection, can thus be very frustrating, both for you and for your doctor. The symptoms of chronic prostatitis are more vague than the symptoms of the acute infection. They can include aching in the area between your scrotum and your rectum, low-back pain, and burning with urination.

Treatment for prostatitis varies. It's easy to control acute bacterial prostatitis with antibiotics, but it's very difficult to completely eradicate it if it develops into the chronic variety. It may require two weeks in some cases, while in others it may take six months. The infection may seemingly disappear, then come back over and over again. In recent years more effective antibiotics have been developed that can penetrate the prostate more successfully, but chronic prostatitis remains a difficult problem to deal with.

Some simple treatments that can help you relieve the symptoms of chronic prostatitis include sitz baths (where the heat seems to have a beneficial effect by increasing blood supply) and prostatic massage, which helps relieve the symptoms by draining fluid from the prostatic ducts.

Zinc also has been thought to play a role in the treatment of chronic prostatitis. Prostatic secretions normally have an antibacterial action that helps to prevent prostate infections. The effectiveness of this antibacterial response has seemed proportional to the levels of zinc in the secretions. Men who have chronic, recurring prostate infections had been thought to have extremely low prostatic zinc levels. More recent studies do not seem to confirm this.

The urologists I consulted say there isn't any definitive scientific evidence that zinc supplementation prevents recurrences of prostatic infections. It does seem to help some men, though, on an empirical and anecdotal basis. Several of my patients have told me that they believe that taking zinc supplements has eliminated recurrences of their chronic prostate infections. Again, though, there is no real proof that this works.

Relatively rarely, chronic prostatitis can cause a peculiar sexual difficulty: Men with this condition may sometimes experience an excruciatingly painful spasm of the prostate muscles when they ejaculate. If a man has a number of painful ejaculations, he may develop difficulty in obtaining erections or ejaculating because of his conditioned reflex against the pain.

CONGESTIVE PROSTATITIS

Another type of prostatitis, called *congestive prostatitis, prostatosis,* or *prostatodynia,* doesn't involve any apparent infection and isn't accompanied by fever or chills. Aside from this, many of the symptoms—frequency, urgency, and inability to start the urinary stream—can resemble the symptoms of infectious prostatitis.

Congestive prostatitis means your prostate is filled with excessive fluid. There are a number of possible causes. First of all, you may have experienced repeated sexual stimulation without ejaculation, causing the production of extra prostatic fluid that hasn't been expelled. (This doesn't mean, however, that you should try to force yourself to ejaculate every time you have sex. Now that you're over forty or fifty, you actually don't have the need to climax each time, because your prostate doesn't make as much prostatic fluid. When your ejaculation fluid builds up, you probably will ejaculate without much difficulty.)

A second possible cause of prostate congestion is constant vibration, which apparently also stimulates the production of prostatic fluid. Motorcyclists and truck drivers, for example, often develop this uncomfortable congestion.

Third, some doctors feel that BPH, or prostatic enlargement, may encourage prostatic congestion by making it difficult for prostatic fluid to drain.

Finally, prostatic congestion can develop in some men without any known cause.

Prostatic congestion can be relieved by ejaculation. A substitute for this is prostatic massage, which milks the excess fluid out of the prostate gland. Hot sitz baths can help with this form of prostatitis, too, and anti-inflammatory agents such as Naproxen can also be of help.

The symptoms of all types of prostatitis, as well as BPH, can suddenly worsen if you eat large amounts of very spicy foods, drink large amounts of coffee or alcohol, or sit on a cold surface for a long time.

Neither infectious nor congestive prostatitis increases your chances of getting cancer of the prostate or of getting BPH, as far as anyone knows.

CANCER OF THE PROSTATE

Cancer is a frightening word, but cancer of the prostate is a very variable illness. Although it sometimes can be quite malignant, often it is slow growing, so that if it is diagnosed early enough it can be treated successfully and even cured.

Prostatic cancer is found primarily in older men. Therefore, as the average life span gets longer, we are seeing more and more of it. While rarely seen in men under forty, by eighty it's fairly common.

If your father had cancer of the prostate, your risk is increased. Black men also seem to be at increased risk. The only dietary factor that seems verified is that a low-fat diet is safer than a high-fat one.

Prostate cancer usually starts in a part of the prostate that is away from the urinary tract, so it rarely causes the kinds of early-warning symptoms that would alert you. But it is extremely important to diagnose prostate cancer early. One of my urology consultants told me that more than half the patients he sees with cancer of the prostate have waited until it's inoperable before coming in. Most of them could have been diagnosed much earlier and probably cured if only they had come in for regular rectal exams. Need I say more?

PROSTATE CANCER TREATMENTS

If the prostate cancer is localized, the best and most common treatment is total *surgical removal.* It has the highest cure rate. It is also the easiest to monitor after surgery.

Unfortunately, however, surgery often damages the nerves involved in obtaining an erection, even in the best of hands. There tends to be about a 25 percent rate of impotence postsurgery and about a 5 percent risk of incontinence.

External Beam Radiation is sometimes used if the patient prefers it or if he is too debilitated to undergo surgery safely. It has a cure rate less than that of surgery and more complications. The impotence rate is as much as 50 percent, and there is a small but significant danger of permanent, very unpleasant, injury to the rectum or bladder from the radiation.

Interstitial Radiation or Brachytherapy involves the implantation of radioactive "seeds" right where they need to go, exactly in the tumor. This method is experiencing a resurgence now that the technology has improved. As the radiation goes exactly where you want it, it spares the rectum and bladder and has a low complication rate. Early reports indicate that it also has a high cure rate.

Hormonal Treatment One way to treat cancer of the prostate is to reduce the amount of testosterone that the body produces, since testosterone may stimulate a prostate cancer. This is sometimes accomplished by giving medication that suppresses testosterone production. In other cases, testosterone is reduced by surgically removing both testicles from the scrotum. The latter, called orchiectomy, is simple and much cheaper than continuing medication, but some men don't like to think of losing their testicles.

Hormonal treatment doesn't cure the cancer, but it makes the patient more comfortable. It is usually used for older patients who already have less than a ten-year life expectancy because of other major health problems.

Since many cancers of the prostate are very slow growing, some people recommend just *observation*, with no treatment, for slow-growing cancers in older men who have a short life expectancy. They feel that these men will probably die of something else before they ever die from the cancer, and it spares them the side effects of treatment. There are quite divided opinions about this, as you would expect.

The *best treatment* for prostate cancer—and the one most likely to spare sexual function—is, of course, treatment performed early in the course of the disease. It's therefore important to have any urinary problems diagnosed early and to have regular rectal exams if you're over forty—probably yearly exams if you're over fifty.

CONTINUING YOUR SEXUAL LIFE
AFTER PROSTATE SURGERY

There is really no reason for prostate problems to end your sexual life. Even if surgery is involved, chances are great that you will retain your erection ability. But if you do not, there are treatments available that will still allow you and your partner to continue to enjoy lovemaking indefinitely.

In a later chapter I will describe the use of penile implants. An implant will allow you to have an erection and to continue to enjoy lovemaking even if you've lost your erection ability due to surgery. If you still have partial ability, Viagra alone may restore your erections without an implant.

CHAPTER 22

TESTOSTERONE

The Hormone of Sexuality

Testosterone is the most active and powerful of the androgen hormones—the masculinizing, or male, hormones, produced by the testes and the adrenal glands. It regulates the development of male sexual features in young boys and teenagers, and it maintains male sexual features in later life. Testosterone also stimulates growth, the production of protein, muscular development, and the deposition of calcium in bones. In addition, testosterone plays a very important role in regulating sexual performance and desire. In fact, testosterone seems to be the hormone most responsible for sexual drive, sexual interest, and sexual responsiveness—in women as well as men.

How, as a male hormone, can testosterone affect sexual desire in women? While androgens are considered to be male sexual hormones, they are actually produced in men and women alike and seem to control sexual desire in both.

Androgens are produced in the adrenal glands of both sexes in approximately equal amounts. They then travel in the bloodstream to the liver, where they're converted into testosterone.

Women's bodies are more responsive to low levels of testosterone, so the relatively small amount of testosterone that women produce is adequate to produce sexual responsiveness for them. The male body, however, requires much more of this hormone. Men produce large additional amounts of it in their testicles, while women's ovaries are producing equally large amounts of the feminizing hormone, estrogen. The extra testosterone that men produce in their testicles results in men having ten to twenty times more testosterone than women have.

Testosterone plays a major part in determining a man's levels of sexual desire, his ability to get an erection, and probably his ability to ejaculate as well. And it has a special significance to an older man, because the amount produced gradually decreases throughout his life, and this loss inevitably plays some role in the diminished sexual appetite and sexual response that may be experienced with aging.

Many factors go into a man's sexual response besides testesterone, of course, including how much attraction you have to your partner, the sexual excitement of the situation, the absence of stress and anxiety, your erection reflex, the blood supply to your penis, and, finally, how directly your penis is stimulated. Unquestionably, though, a true deficiency of testosterone will interfere with the quality of your erections, even if all other circumstances are ideal.

WHAT CAN TESTOSTERONE
REPLACEMENT DO?

Can testosterone reverse problems of loss of sexual desire, erection ability, and ability to ejaculate? When it first became available, doctors used testosterone to treat any man who came along complaining of impotence. The results were generally disappointing, because in any group of impotent men only a small minority have testosterone deficiency as the sole cause.

If you're experiencing these problems and your testosterone level is *clearly deficient*, testosterone replacement is worth a try. In cases of deficiency it can produce a striking and dramatic improvement. It is especially helpful in treating *lack of desire* in men with deficient testosterone levels. It can also produce a marked improvement in one's *sense of well-being*.

Unfortunately, however, even if your testosterone levels are deficient, hormone replacement isn't guaranteed to correct impotence, since erection difficulties have many possible causes. If nerve damage or blocked blood vessels, for example, are the cause of your problem, all the testosterone in the world won't facilitate erections.

WHO SHOULD TRY TESTOSTERONE?

Many doctors feel that testosterone should be restricted to men who have clearly deficient levels and loss of desire. My own inclinations are somewhat different. If a man of sixty with erection problems and some loss of desire has a "low normal" testosterone level, he may indeed still be within the "normal" range for a man in his sixties, but it's certainly much lower than the level he had when he was in his twenties. As his erection mechanism has become more fragile with age, he may now be on the border between getting erections or not getting them. The extra boost that restoring his testosterone level can give him may be all he needs to restore libido and to get him functioning again.

I have observed that many older men respond favorably to testosterone when their hormone levels are in the lower range of what is considered normal, especially when the hormone is prescribed in conjunction with other erection-improving medications.

HOW IS TESTOSTERONE PRESCRIBED?

Clearly, testosterone has potential in restoring sexual vigor and desire for at least some older men. Let's review how it is administered.

Testosterone ordinarily has a brief life in the body, since it is broken down rapidly in the liver. Additional testosterone taken orally isn't very effective, as it is quickly digested and destroyed. For this reason, longer-acting forms of testosterone were developed, combining the hormone chemically in order to slow its breakdown in your body. Methyltestosterone is one of the longer-acting forms that is not metabolized as rapidly as is plain testosterone. At one time this was a form that was given *orally*, but it is no longer used for men because the doses required for them posed a danger of liver toxicity.

Most experts believe that the oral administration of methyltestosterone wasn't as effective, in any case, as *injections* of still-longer-acting forms such as testosterone cypionate and testosterone enanthate, which are now used. In men who are testosterone deficient, an injection of 300 to 400 milligrams of testosterone enanthate once a month will usually be quite effective. For some men, however, the dose won't last for a full month, and others feel high or even aggressive at first and then feel flat in the last half of the month. For these reasons 200 milligrams every two to three weeks will give better and more even results in many cases, with more stable hormone levels.

If getting to a doctor every two to four weeks is a problem, you can learn to administer the shots yourself. Or, because the shots are usually administered in the buttocks, it may be easier to have your partner give them to you.

After testosterone injections begin, a previously hormone-deficient man will probably notice some improvement in his erection ability within two weeks. Some men don't really feel the full benefit of the treatment until the second injection, when the hormone level has been built up.

More recently, testosterone *skin patches* in different strengths have been introduced. They need to be replaced once a day. The testosterone is absorbed through the skin directly into the bloodstream. This means that it doesn't have to be in a methyl compound like the oral compounds or in a cyprionate or enanthate compound like the injectable forms. This may make it safer to use.

The first patches to come out were worn on the scrotum. It was necessary to shave an area on the scrotum where the patch was to be applied. More recently patches have been introduced that can be worn on the back or upper arm. Most men prefer these, although it may be necessary to shave these places too before application.

It will probably take several weeks for full effectiveness after starting use of the testosterone patches.

To compare the two methods: The advantages of the injections are that they cost less and they have to be administered only once every few weeks instead of replaced daily like the patch. The disadvantages of the injections are first that they are injections, which some people don't like, and second that they don't give a consistent blood level over the three or four weeks but cause a peak during which the patient may feel more aggressive and then a trough in blood level during which the patient may feel apathetic. Again, this can be partly overcome by giving the shots every two weeks as described above.

The advantages of the patches are that they give a more consistent blood level and that they don't require a shot. The disadvantages are that they require daily applications and they can cause local skin irritation such as rash or itching at the site of application. Some men comment that although the patches seem to work, they don't feel quite as effective as the shots.

To overcome some of these objections, *testosterone gels and creams* are under development. These may eliminate the irrritation at the application sites and will also not be visible to one's partner as the patch is. They are not yet on the market, though.

POSSIBLE SIDE EFFECTS

Besides its benefit to sexual activity, testosterone has other actions, some of which can cause undesirable side effects for a small number of men. The vast majority, however, will probably never experience any of the possible side effects listed below.

Testosterone may cause the kidneys to increase the amount of water and salt they retain. This rarely causes problems, though, except when the hormone is administered in extremely large doses, or if you already have kidney or liver trouble or congestive heart failure.

Salt and water retention can also cause trouble if you have high blood pressure, migraine headaches, or epilepsy. With the usual dose of testosterone replacement, however, it is unlikely that enough salt and water will be retained to cause difficulty, even if you have one of these conditions.

Testosterone stimulates red blood cell production, so that large doses conceivably could cause excessive production of red blood cells, a rare condition known as polycythemia. In addition, testosterone increases blood levels of calcium, but not usually by amounts that are clinically significant.

Another property of testosterone is that it stimulates the sebaceous glands, which theoretically could cause acne. Nevertheless, I have yet to see acne produced in an older man by testosterone replacement.

Some testosterone is changed into estrogen during its breakdown. Therefore, if large amounts are given, some breast enlargement due to the increased estrogen might possibly occur.

Testosterone also stimulates the cells of the prostate gland. For this reason, men taking it require regular checkups for signs of prostatic enlargement, and *those men with cancer of the prostate must avoid it altogether*, because it could stimulate the growth of that type of cancer cells. It is not believed, however, that testosterone will cause a prostate cancer if there isn't one there to begin with. Although it is unlikely that you have cancer of the prostate, for safety's sake it's important to have your prostate checked before starting testosterone treatment, and periodically while you are taking it.

In rare cases, testosterone causes excessive sexual stimulation and painful erections that won't recede, a condition known as priapism.

Very large doses of testosterone can send a false message to your pituitary gland that your testicles are putting out plenty of hormones. Your pituitary gland will therefore produce fewer of the hormones that ordinarily stimulate your testicles. This can result in a lowered sperm count, which may cause difficulty if a couple is trying to conceive. Large doses of testosterone may also cause some decrease in the size of your testicles, as they will have less work to do.

Diabetics receiving testosterone may have to adjust their dosage of insulin or oral hypoglycemic medicine, since testosterone may slightly alter their capacity to handle sugar.

IN SUMMARY

If you are over forty, your levels of testosterone have gradually decreased over the years. The slide began when you were about twenty years old. Some men in their fifties, sixties, and seventies still have adequate levels of testesterone, but others do not. These lower hormone levels may be associated with loss of desire, loss of potency, loss of ability to climax, and loss of ejaculatory ability.

If your hormone levels are deficient, the administration of testosterone may rapidly and strikingly restore sexual desire and erection ability. But it must be emphasized that there are many other causes for sexual dysfunction, and testosterone will only provide the answer for a minority of men.

Finally, testosterone can bring with it some possible serious side effects. How you might be affected will depend on your own unique medical condition and history. A thorough examination by, and discussion with, your own physician is therefore imperative before beginning any testosterone replacement.

CHAPTER 23

WILL A HYSTERECTOMY AFFECT YOUR SEXUAL LIFE?

It's estimated that more than half of all women in the United States will have a hysterectomy by age sixty-five. It's one of the most common major operations performed in the United States. Theoretically, a hysterectomy should have little or no effect on a woman's sexual life, but unfortunately, for some, it does cause major problems.

You might expect that information about the sexual side effects of hysterectomy would be clear-cut and readily available, but this isn't the case. There is a lot of controversy, and experts on the subject frequently contradict one another. What follows is the best understanding I can give you. It's based on my evaluation of many often conflicting studies and on my years of clinical practice.

WHAT IS A HYSTERECTOMY?

Let's start off by defining the terms that we'll be using:

Hysterectomy   refers to the removal of your *uterus* (or womb), an organ about the size of a pear that is located at the end of your vaginal canal. During pregnancy, the fertilized egg attaches itself to the uterine lining, and the fetus grows inside the uterus. Monthly menstrual periods are the shedding of the lining of the uterus when it has not been used for pregnancy.

The part of your uterus that protrudes into the far end of your vagina is called your *cervix*. The cervix is removed along with the rest of your uterus during a *total hysterectomy* (usually just referred to as a "hysterectomy"). A hysterectomy will end your menstrual periods if you're still having them, since menstrual bleeding comes from your uterus. It will also mean that you can no longer get pregnant. Your ovaries, however, will continue to produce hormones in a cyclical fashion. When that comes to a stop, you go through *menopause.*

Sometimes, during a hysterectomy, the ovaries are removed as well. Removal of your ovaries is called an *oophorectomy*. It produces a "surgical menopause" if you have not already been through menopause anyway. That's because the removal of the source of estrogen causes a sudden, sharp drop in hormonal levels in your body. This may cause such marked withdrawal symptoms as hot flashes, anxiety, and irritability. Estrogen replacement therapy is usually advised (see chapter 4 on estrogen replacement).

A hysterectomy is customarily performed in one of two ways. In a *vaginal hysterectomy*, the surgery is performed through the vagina and leaves no external scar. An *abdominal hysterectomy* is usually performed with a "bikini incision" in the abdomen just above the pubic area.

The vaginal approach is preferable if it is indicated, because it causes less trauma and there is a quicker recovery. However, an abdominal approach is usually necessary if the ovaries have to be removed, if there is a large tumor or cyst, or if postmenopausal lack of estrogen has caused vaginal shrinkage. Abdominal hysterectomies are actually more common.

Recovery from an abdominal hysterectomy usually requires about two to three days in the hospital, whereas a laparoscopy-assisted, vaginal hysterectomy usually requires about one day of hospitalization. It usually takes about four to six weeks before you can return to full activity.

It's important to keep in mind that the sexual and reproductive organs and functions aren't the same, although they sometimes work together. A hysterectomy removes your uterus, which is primarily a reproductive organ. It doesn't affect your vagina, your clitoris, or your labia, which are your primary sexual organs.

WHY ARE HYSTERECTOMIES PERFORMED?

Some common causes of hysterectomy for premenopausal women include irregular uterine bleeding or prolonged periods, endometriosis, uterine myomas, and pelvic inflammatory disease.

Older women are more likely to require hysterectomy for postmenopausal bleeding or for cancerous or precancerous conditions of the uterus, and occasionally still for fibroids.

Uterine prolapse, or sagging of the uterus into the vagina, is a common cause for hysterectomy in women of any age who have had several children.

WILL I LOSE MY FEMININITY?

There are some terrifying myths regarding the aftereffects of a hysterectomy. They may leave a woman facing a hysterectomy with unreasonable worries about what will happen to her after the operation, in addition to the anxiety that normally precedes any surgery.

Many of these fears are based on misconceptions about what a hysterectomy actually involves. Louise D., whom I recently treated, became very depressed after surgery and felt that she was "cleaned out and empty inside," that she had somehow lost her femininity and desirability. Other women worry that they will suddenly become overweight or prematurely aged.

Many apprehensions about hysterectomy are, of course, specifically related to a woman's sexual life. She may worry that hysterectomy will end her sexual life entirely, or else cause her to lose her attractiveness, her sexual desire, or her ability to satisfy her partner sexually.

Let's examine the facts. When you're aware of the relatively small size of your nonpregnant uterus (about the size and shape of a pear, as I mentioned before), it will be clear to you that you won't be "empty" after a hysterectomy. There is no medical reason for you to suddenly gain weight or to lose your attractiveness. A hysterectomy doesn't end your sexual life. It should have no effect at all on your ability to satisfy your partner sexually, and in most cases it won't have any effect on your sexual desire.

WHAT CAN I ACTUALLY EXPECT
AFTER A HYSTERECTOMY?

There is a wide range of medical opinions about the effects of a hysterectomy. At one end of the spectrum, authorities claim that a hysterectomy should not cause any emotional or sexual problems at all. At the other extreme, a few studies report that one-third of all women who have undergone the operation suffer a "posthysterectomy syndrome," with depression and loss of sexual desire for several months afterward.

Actually, reports of the posthysterectomy syndrome's depression and loss of sexual desire seem greatly exaggerated. A few weeks of fatigue and emotionality, which may follow any major stress or surgery, are not abnormal after hysterectomy. However, most studies show women to have improved mood and energy, as well as unimpaired sexual desire and sexual response, when they are evaluated several months after the operation.

One study that examined women both before and after their hysterectomy, for example, reported that 90 percent described themselves as pleased, and 85 percent would encourage a friend to have the procedure performed. Only 4 percent said that they felt worse. Those women who were depressed following the operation generally turned out to have been depressed before as well.

Your expectations before a hysterectomy are a very important factor in how you'll feel after it. If you believe that you will lose your femininity, that your partner will no longer desire you, or that you'll lose your own sexual desire, you're more likely to become depressed and to have actual sexual difficulty after the operation. On the other hand, if you look forward to the operation as a way of getting rid of uncomfortable symptoms such as bleeding, urinary incontinence, or painful intercourse, you are likely to feel pleased after the operation and to have undiminished sexual desire.

If your cultural or religious background stresses that pregnancy is the only legitimate reason for sex and that nonfertile women are therefore not considered sexual, you may be more likely to have sexual difficulty. If you strongly desire more children, if you have had depressions before in response to stress, or if you have had many recurrent or chronic physical complaints, you may possibly have trouble after the operation.

Even if you are an over-forty woman who had no plans at all of having any more children, you may feel a special sense of loss at the finality of hysterectomy. This is especially so if part of what makes you feel feminine is caught up with the *potential* of being a mother and having babies.

The support and encouragement of your partner is very important. Reassurance that he continues to find you sexual and appealing after your hysterectomy will go a long way toward making your response a positive one.

If you do continue to feel depressed after a hysterectomy, be sure to get the necessary psychiatric care. It can make a tremendous difference.

WILL MY SEXUAL LIFE CONTINUE?

Almost all women who were sexually active before a hysterectomy continue to be sexually active afterward. At least 80 percent resume sexual relations within eight weeks following surgery, although more than half feel some mild discomfort at first.

HOW SHOULD I RESUME INTERCOURSE?

Your gynecologist will probably want to see you about one month after the operation. At this time, he or she will check the back of your vagina to make sure it's completely healed and give you the okay to begin lovemaking.

It's natural to have some apprehension and soreness when you first make love following surgery. Your apprehension can cause lack of vaginal lubrication at first and even some involuntary flinching or constriction of your vaginal opening.

Remember that your clitoris and labia were not affected by the surgery. They shouldn't be tender, and you should enjoy clitoral stimulation. Because anxiety can cause lack of lubrication, it's best to use a sexual lubricant such as Astroglide at first.

Your partner can help you get used to sex again in a gradual way. Suggest to him that you would like him to stimulate your clitoris, manually or orally. This will help you to get your own natural lubrication back and will help to restore your sexual confidence. Then tell him that you would like to guide first his finger and then his penis into your vagina in a controlled way, and ask that he not do any thrusting until you're sure that you feel comfortable.

You might start with the female superior position, in which you kneel over your partner's hips. You'll feel more in control and more secure in this position. Begin by inserting your partner's penis just partway into your vagina. As you become reassured that it's not painful, you will start to enjoy the feeling of his penis in your vagina again. You can then choose when to continue to full intercourse. If discomfort continues in spite of your precautions, consult with your gynecologist about it.

WHAT ABOUT THE PROBLEM
OF "DRY VAGINA"?

Some women report lack of vaginal lubrication following a hysterectomy. This should be a temporary problem if it's due to anxiety and apprehension. But, if your hysterectomy included the removal of your ovaries, the loss of estrogens can cause a lasting lack of lubrication.

Using a sexual lubricant or lovemaking oil is a simple solution. Estrogen replacement therapy will also help to rapidly restore your vaginal lubrication and to maintain the health of your vaginal tissue. (Again, see our chapter on estrogen replacement.)

WHAT EFFECT WILL THERE BE
ON MY SEXUAL DESIRE?

Most women, probably 75 percent of them, find that their level of sexual desire is unaffected by a hysterectomy. Perhaps 20 percent report that they have more sexual desire after the hysterectomy, probably because sexual discomfort or other gynecologic symptoms were eliminated by the surgery.

On the other hand, a small minority of women definitely report some decrease of sexual desire. The few I've seen with this problem all had had their ovaries removed as well as their uteruses.

Theoretically, this drop in sexual desire shouldn't occur. The androgen hormones that regulate sexual desire are produced primarily by the adrenals in women and shouldn't be affected by removing either the uterus or the ovaries. However, most of women's testosterone, which is the most active androgen, is produced by the ovaries. Removal of the ovaries may thus cause a fall in testosterone levels, and this may produce a loss of sexual desire.

Administering testosterone to a woman who has experienced loss of sexual desire following a hysterectomy and oophorectomy will very likely restore her desire. Estrogen alone can restore vaginal lubrication and prevent atrophy, but it has little or no effect on reestablishing sexual desire. It has therefore been suggested that estrogen replacement therapy for postmenopausal and posthysterectomy women should regularly include a small amount of testosterone to maintain a feeling of well-being and sexual desire. Even if a woman can't take estrogens for medical reasons, she may be able to take testosterone safely.

WILL I ENJOY INTERCOURSE?
WILL I STILL BE ABLE TO CLIMAX?

Many women report that they find intercourse more enjoyable after a hysterectomy, especially if they were having physical discomfort before the operation. Many more women find their level of enjoyment essentially unchanged, while only a very few, perhaps 5 percent or less, report diminished enjoyment.

A small but definite group of women report a distinct change in the character of their orgasm, or difficulty in achieving orgasm, after a hysterectomy. Why this should be so is not immediately obvious, because for most women the stimulus for orgasm is either the clitoris or a vaginal trigger-point such as the G-spot. These areas are usually not affected by the operation.

For those women who develop difficulty postoperatively, however, the orgasm was apparently triggered by the thrusting of their partner's penis against their cervix and uterus. They experienced orgasm deep within their pelvis and may now have considerable difficulty achieving orgasm since the cervix and uterus have been removed. It may be necessary for such a woman to learn to climax with clitoral stimulation. This is not necessarily an unpleasant prospect, but it will require some rethinking and relearning and an acceptance that her responses are now different.

WILL A HYSTERECTOMY CAUSE ME TO ENTER MENOPAUSE?

If you've not yet begun menopause, the removal of your ovaries will cause you to enter menopause immediately. Even if your ovaries are left behind, however, a hysterectomy may occasionally precipitate an early menopause. This occurs within one to two years after surgery for some women. The reason that this happens is not clear, but if it does occur you should consider estrogen replacement therapy strongly, as women who have an early menopause are prime candidates for osteoporosis, cardiovascular disease, and the other symptoms of chronic estrogen deprivation that we discussed in an earlier chapter.

PART

5

OVERCOMING ERECTION DIFFICULTIES

CHAPTER 24

HOW TO EVALUATE
YOUR ERECTION PROBLEMS

I have already discussed how a man experiences an inevitable slowdown in his sexual drive and his sexual ability as he ages. It's a rare man who continues, at age fifty-five or sixty, to have the same sexual appetite that he had when he was twenty or twenty-five. But in spite of these changes, your sexual life can actually become more satisfying as you develop more skills, more appreciation of your own sensuality and that of your partner, and more feeling of sexual contentment.

Unfortunately, not every older man experiences this increased enjoyment. For many older men, the slowdown becomes a stop. Erections may become infrequent, too soft for penetration, or nonexistent.

This can be one of the most humiliating experiences an older man may have to endure. Most men don't know where to go for help, and they are often too embarrassed to ask for it, in any case.

Well, there have been enormous advances in the treatment of erection problems, and there *is* help available now.

ERECTION DIFFICULTY IS A VERY COMMON PROBLEM

In my practice I saw many, many men with concerns about erection ability, and each case presented a number of possibilities that had to be investigated. Some men suffer from impotence due to medical illness, vascular insufficiency, hormonal deficiencies, or medication side effects. Others have erection difficulty due to anxiety about their functioning, pressure from their partner, stress, or relationship difficulties. Still others have no real erection problems at all but are frightened by some of the normal sexual changes that come with aging.

Emotional and physical factors often interact to add to a man's difficulty. If he is experiencing minor changes in his sexual responses—due to vascular insufficiency, for instance—and he becomes frightened by them, his anxiety can cause him to have much more trouble getting hard than he would have had otherwise. Anxiety about performance can thus magnify the sexual difficulty that a medical condition may be causing.

Over the years, I have compiled a list of questions that help me to assess whether a patient's erection problems are primarily medical or emotional. They also give me some clues as to what the specific problem is. You can ask yourself the same questions before going to your personal physician.

The answers you get will give you at least a preliminary idea of what's wrong. In addition, not every doctor you may consult may know very much about sexual problems, so your own preliminary evaluation may help you to judge whether the physician has a reasonable grasp of the problem.

DO YOU NOT GET ERECTIONS AT ALL, OR DO YOU GET THEM BUT THEN LOSE THEM?

This seems like a simple question, but my interpretation of your answer depends in part on my experience in treating hundreds of men with these problems.

If, for example, you tell me that a few years ago you gradually began to lose your erections more and more easily and that now you don't get any erections at all, chances are you have a slowly developing physical problem. If you get erections that are terrific until you try to penetrate but then rapidly go down just as you enter your partner, your problem is probably due to anxiety about your performance. If your erection comes up halfway or three-quarters with a lot of stimulation but then goes right back down as soon as the stimulation ends, it's more likely to be a physical problem. If your erection comes up normally but then fades during intercourse, it could mean that the blood is leaking out of your erection and back into your general body circulation. If, on the other hand, you are able to have intercourse for a good while, perhaps ten or fifteen minutes, but then your erection sometimes fades away, there's probably nothing wrong with you at all. One erection doesn't have to stay forever. If it goes down, your partner can probably help you get it back. If you don't climax on a particular occasion, it probably just means that your body doesn't need a climax at that time.

DO YOU OCCASIONALLY AWAKEN
WITH A FIRM ERECTION?

This is a good way to tell whether your erectile mechanism has the
capacity to function. If it does, you will, during the course of an
ordinary night's sleep, have three or four erections lasting approx-
mately twenty minutes each. These occur during the stage of
sleep called REM sleep, or dream sleep. You may not be aware of
the erections while you're asleep, but if you happen to awaken
during this stage of sleep you will be likely to awaken with an
erection.

If you awaken with a full bladder, that's *not* the cause of the
erection. It's just that your urge to urinate happened to wake you
up during a dream-sleep stage.

If you do notice fairly regular middle-of-the-night or morning erections, it's a good indication that your erection mechanism is intact and does have the capacity to function. If you are
aware of erections on awakening only very infrequently or not at
all, or if they are very soft erections, it doesn't necessarily prove
that your erection mechanism isn't working—you just may not be
waking up during the appropriate stage of sleep—but it certainly
does raise suspicions that your erection mechanism may be impaired.

CAN YOU GET ERECT IN SOME
SITUATIONS BUT NOT IN OTHERS?

This is a good way to tell whether your erection difficulty is due
to the particular circumstances of your lovemaking or if there's a
medical problem. For example, having difficulty getting erect

when you're very fatigued or under a lot of emotional stress is fairly normal. If, on the other hand, you have problems getting erect with one partner but not another, it may be due to tension that you're feeling in one of the relationships, or it may be that with one partner you feel secure but with the other you feel a lot of pressure to perform. It may even be that one partner helps you get hard and the other doesn't. If erection difficulties occur only with new partners, it's probably because you feel anxiety about your sexual performance in these situations. If you can get erections when you're away on vacation but have difficulty when you're at home, your difficulty may be due to work-related stress.

DOES YOUR PARTNER HELP BY STIMULATING YOUR PENIS? DOES IT WORK WHEN SHE DOES?

This is really an important question. If you haven't been getting help from your partner, it may turn out that there is nothing wrong with you at all. As you get older, you are simply not going to be getting spontaneous erections the way you did when you were younger. You require some direct physical stimulation to your penis in order to get hard. If your partner isn't helping you because she doesn't realize your need for it or because she has left-over inhibitions about touching your penis, your trouble may be due simply to lack of stimulation.

If you can get good erections when your partner stimulates you, there is nothing wrong with your erection mechanism at all. There's nothing unusual or abnormal about requiring stimulation. You and your partner simply need to use foreplay regularly before attempting intercourse.

On the other hand, if you don't get erect even with adequate stimulation, either a medical condition could be causing the problem, or anxiety could be blocking your natural sexual response.

CAN YOU GET ERECT WITH MASTURBATION?

If you can get firm erections with masturbation, your sexual response system is intact. Masturbation when you're alone allows you to try out your erection mechanism in a situation with less anxiety about performance and less embarrassment.

If you have difficulty getting erect during lovemaking, even with some stimulation, but you can get erect with masturbation, there are two possibilities. One is that anxieties about getting hard, or other emotional feelings such as anger or resentment, are blocking your sexual response. The other possibility is that your partner isn't giving you the kind of sexual stimulation that you need. This could be because you've never told her what you'd like or shown her explicitly how to do it. Talking about it might be a little embarrassing, but it can really help.

DID YOUR ERECTION DIFFICULTY START WITH A PARTICULAR, EMOTIONALLY UPSETTING EXPERIENCE?

If your problem started around the time of a divorce or separation, the loss of a job, your retirement, a period of financial stress, the death of your spouse, rejection by your partner, or any similar stressful situation, your erection difficulty was probably a natural response to stress. It may, however, have caused you to worry about your erection ability. If your erection problem has continued past the stress period, it could be that this performance anxiety has continued to interfere.

ARE YOU DEPRESSED?

Depression is a common cause of sexual dysfunction. If you've been feeling sad, discouraged, and lacking in energy, with sleep or appetite disturbances, your sexual problem could simply be another symptom of your depression.

This type of erection problem usually responds very well to appropriate antidepressant medication. Although occasionally patients have sexual side effects from some of these medications, most do not, and overcoming the depression will result in enough liberation of your sexual ability as to outweigh any sexual side effects in most cases anyway!

HOW DO YOU REACT IF YOU HAVE
TROUBLE GETTING HARD?
HOW DOES YOUR PARTNER REACT?

If you tell me your partner becomes angry, accusing, or tearful if you don't get erect, I know that you must feel very pressured to perform. If you become angry or disgusted with yourself if things go wrong, you put the same pressure on yourself.

On the other hand, if your partner is supportive and helpful and you yourself are philosophical but, even so, you have trouble getting hard, there would seem to be less likelihood of your erection difficulty being caused by anxiety alone, and a greater possibility that medical factors might be to blame.

ARE YOU TAKING A MEDICINE THAT
COULD CAUSE ERECTION DIFFICULTIES?

As discussed in previous chapters, many medications can cause erection difficulties. The most prominent of these are the antihypertensives, but many other types of medicines, both mentioned and not included in this book, occasionally cause problems. Review any medicine you might be taking, and check with your own physician if you have a question.

Remember, if you are taking a medication that has been known to occasionally cause sexual difficulties, this doesn't necessarily prove that that medication is the cause of *YOUR* problem. There are many other possible causes for erection difficulties.

HOW YOUR DOCTOR WILL
EVALUATE THE PROBLEM

The questions above will give you some idea of the possible causes of your difficulty. Remember, however, that a comprehensive medical evaluation is necessary to more accurately pin down the exact problem, to rule out more serious illness (such as diabetes) that could be causing it, and to define a treatment plan.

Not too many years ago, impotence was thought to be psychologically caused in almost all cases, because we simply didn't have the means of medically evaluating the problem. The first step toward a fuller understanding came when tests were developed to help distinguish between medical and psychological causes. Then a radical new development was introduced: penile implants to surgically treat impotent men. Soon the pendulum swung the other way. Men with impotence were no longer told that it was all in their heads. Instead, they were being told that surgery was their only hope.

Progress has continued in the past few years. Developments in medical pharmacology and technology have provided a wide spectrum of investigative tools and treatment methods to help men with impotence.

Unfortunately, many who claim to treat impotence are still years behind. Some nonmedical "sexual therapists" still attempt to treat impotent men with sexual counseling alone—ignoring all we have learned in recent years about the medical causes of the problem. Others, like some physicians, still think only in terms of implant surgery for every impotent man. This is also completely unwarranted. Penile implants work extremely well when they are needed, but there are now many other means of treatment that don't require surgery. Automatically recommending surgery, without seeing whether a man's erectile mechanism can be improved by simple medical means, is outmoded and unjustified.

The first step in an evaluation will be to ask the same questions that you asked yourself, above. These will help the doctor determine if the problem is a physical one or primarily due to anxiety. Problems due to anxiety are just as real, of course. If you can't get erect, you can't get erect—whatever the cause. It's also important to determine whether the problem is due primarily to a lack of physical stimulation, which can readily be remedied.

Whether your erection mechanism is intact can be determined by your ability to get erections with masturbation and/or whether you awaken with erections. If you can tell me that you wake up several mornings a week with a good, hard erection, I know that you are getting good nocturnal erections. Further tests to demonstrate this are unnecessary, and a waste of your time and money. If, on the other hand, you don't seem to get nighttime erections, it may be worthwhile to investigate further.

There is a test to examine your nighttime erections called the Nocturnal Penile Tumescence test (NPT). It usually requires that you spend three nights in a sleep lab or hospital, however. Because of the expense and inconvenience of the NPT test, there was a search for simpler, less expensive ways to measure nighttime erections.

One amazingly simple but ingenious variation, the "stamp test," uses a ring of postage stamps placed around the shaft of your penis. If you obtain a full erection, your erection should split the perforations. This test is subject to errors and inexactness, but it's a good first approximation. If you break the stamps three nights out of three, it certainly indicates that your erection mechanism is functioning.

Another test, the "snap-gauge," consists of a Velcro band slipped around your penis. It has three tiny plastic threads, and if your penis gets hard enough for vaginal penetration, all three threads theoretically will break.

Usually these tests of nighttime erection are used only for supplementary evidence because they don't really affect the treatment. We usually have a good idea whether or not you are awakening with firm erections from your own report. We also know that almost all of our older patients will have at least some physical or vascular component to their erection problem anyway.

All in all, tests of nighttime erections must be interpreted with caution. If you get no nighttime erections, it's usually a good indication that you have a physical problem. However, I'm not sure that getting a reflex erection in your sleep necessarily proves that you should be able to get hard in a sexual situation or that the problem is "in your head."

COULD A SUBSTANCE YOU ARE TAKING BE AFFECTING YOUR SEXUAL FUNCTIONING?

The antihypertensive medications are the most likely culprits, but there are many other possibilities. Because your high blood pressure, if you have it, needs to be treated, your physician will search for a medication that will control that problem without suppressing your sexual functioning. It's the same with medications you may be taking for other illnesses.

Long-term overuse of alcohol and cigarettes causes major sexual problems for many of the older men who come to the clinic. Remember, amounts of alcohol that presented no problem when you were in your twenties may be enough to overwhelm your erection reflex now that you are older and your erections have become more fragile. Likewise, smoking can be an erection killer.

Chronic use of marijuana or cocaine can suppress sexual function. Opiates like heroin will wipe it out. Chronic use of steroids for muscle building will shrink your testicles and decrease your testosterone.

COULD AN ILLNESS BE AFFECTING YOU SEXUALLY?

To start off with the obvious, surgery or radiation treatment for prostate cancer can damage the nerves leading to the penis, as can any traumatic accident in that area.

Then, your doctor will especially look for arteriosclerosis, high blood pressure, diabetes, hormonal problems, or chronic liver or kidney dysfunction.

Diabetes stands out as a frequent cause of erection problems. Many men who have had this disease for some time develop a decreased erection ability, either because of neuropathy (nerve damage) or vascular damage (partial blockage of the blood supply to the penis). Some men we see for erection difficulties don't realize that they have diabetes, while others have known about it for years but often have not taken good care of themselves.

Arteriosclerosis, or hardening of the arteries, causes blockage of the small blood vessels leading to the penis the same way that it blocks the blood flow in other parts of the body. Chronic liver disease can alter the ways that sexual hormones are metabolized in the body and result in a relative lack of male hormones.

Hypothyroidism (low thyroid hormone) can also be associated with decreased production and increased breakdown of male hormones. Patients with this condition may have increased production of prolactin, a pituitary hormone that suppresses sexual desire and erection in men. Patients with hypothyroidism may also develop fatigue, lethargy, or depression, all of which may also suppress sexual desire and functioning, but it's usually unlikely that hypothyroidism is the sole cause of a person's erection problems.

We test for these conditions in a number of ways. Laboratory evaluations can be especially helpful. A chemistry profile gives us a blood sugar level to screen for diabetes and also tests various liver and kidney functions. In most cases, we also check thyroid function.

Elevated levels of the hormone prolactin can cause sexual difficulty. Produced by the pituitary gland, its primary function is to stimulate women's breasts to produce milk. While also produced in small quantities in men, it doesn't have any male function that we know of. If too much of it is produced, however, depression of male sexual desire, suppression of testosterone production, and erection difficulty may result.

Various conditions can elevate prolactin levels. One is the presence of a pituitary adenoma, a small, usually nonmalignant tumor, which produces very high levels of this hormone. Other conditions that can cause moderate elevations are hypothyroidism and various medications, such as major tranquilizers. Stress can also contribute. Elevated prolactin levels are uncommon as a cause of impotence, but they certainly do occur. Often, prolactin levels are checked only if your testosterone level is decreased, as elevated prolactin can suppress testosterone.

In another chapter, I discussed at length the role of testosterone, your primary male hormone, in sexual function. As this hormone may be depressed in many older men, testosterone levels are usually checked routinely as part of a work-up.

THE UROLOGICAL EXAM

A urologist will usually check your testicles for signs of atrophy or shrinkage that could indicate inadequate testicular function. A rectal exam will enable him to check your prostate gland for signs of enlargement, infection, or tumor.

Your penis will be examined for any abnormality and especially for signs of Peyronie's disease. This peculiar condition, seen more commonly in older men, results in a fibrous thickening or plaque on the side or top of the penis, which can cause sharp bending of the penis with erection. This can be quite painful. The condition can also create an inability to get erect. Its cause is unknown.

An important part of the urological examination will be a test of your perineal sensation and bulbocavernosal reflex to make sure that the nerves that produce erections are not grossly impaired.

The urologist may also perform a simple test of the blood pressure in your penis and will compare the results with the blood pressure in the rest of your body to help us estimate whether the circulation to your penis has been impaired by arteriosclerosis or other conditions. As with so many other tests dealing with impotence, this one isn't 100 percent certain either. Some men with good blood pressure in their penises still can't get erect, while other men with what seems to be decreased penile blood pressure get fine erections.

When men come to us with erection problems, they occasionally tell us how previous urologists have done huge work-ups, which have included IVPs (kidney evaluations) and cystoscopies (bladder evaluations). In almost all cases, an IVP and cystoscopy are irrelevant in an impotence work-up; there's no reason for you to go through the unnecessary expense and inconvenience of these tests.

IN SUMMARY

This gives you a good idea of how you can evaluate your sexual problem, and how your doctor will evaluate it. We will now give you an idea of how erection problems are treated in the next chapter.

CHAPTER 25

HOW WE TREAT
ERECTION PROBLEMS

A s we described in chapter 2, Viagra has created a true revolution in the treatment of sexual dysfunction, but it is important to realize that there are many problems that can be treated, very easily, *without adding any medication at all.*

IF THE PROBLEM IS DUE TO LACK
OF STIMULATION OR ANXIETY
ABOUT PERFORMANCE

First of all, as we mentioned earlier, one of the easiest problems to treat is simple lack of penile stimulation. Working with you and your partner together makes for the most effective treatment.

Both of you need to realize that an older man usually requires assistance from his partner to get erect. It's time to set aside inhibitions about a woman touching a man's penis so you can continue to have a satisfying sexual life together. Certainly, a medicine like Viagra could help you overcome this, but it's silly to take an expensive medicine if all you need is some stimulation.

If anxiety about performance is adding to your difficulties in getting erect there are two complementary approaches to treatment that your doctor can take. The first would be to involve your partner and explain that her help and cheerful cooperation is necessary. While doing that, the second approach would be to also give you a medication that will help you get erect if all else fails. This could be Viagra or penile injections, for example (more about these later in this chapter).

Once you discover that Viagra or the injection can give you an erection at will, you will likely stop worrying about your erection. Having assurance that you can function will take the pressure off. If anxiety about performance was the primary reason you couldn't function, you will probably be able to get hard most of the time in the future without needing or using the medication, just keeping it in reserve as a backup.

Your partner may well have become frustrated with your erection difficulties, which is certainly understandable, but her frustration can mean additional pressure for you. Your doctor should explain to her that getting upset and criticizing you actually produce a result opposite to the one she wants.

If part of your difficulty is due to fatigue or stress, changing some of the environmental factors in your life would obviously be a good idea. I'd also suggest such simple alternatives as making love in the morning or on the weekend, when you're relaxed and not under pressure.

IF YOUR PROBLEMS ARE DUE
TO MEDICATION OR SUBSTANCE
SIDE EFFECTS

As you know by now, quite a number of frequently used medications can cause loss of sexual desire and erection ability. Because their sexual side effects are not widely publicized, your physician may not be aware of them.

If your doctor discovers that you may be taking one or more medications that could be contributing to your sexual difficulties, he or she should try to advise you of simple alternatives that have less risk of causing these problems. There usually are alternatives.

Often your physician may not be sure that a specific medication is adversely affecting your sexual function. In that case, he or she may suggest strategies to test whether this medication or some other factor is the primary cause.

As we mentioned earlier, excessive alcohol use and cigarette smoking are very common causes of erection difficulty, especially in older men. If either of these circumstances is contributing in a major way to your sexual difficulties, we would strongly urge that you make some alterations in your consumption patterns.

We find that it's relatively easy for men to cut back on their alcohol consumption when they realize that it is causing sexual difficulties. Cigarette smoking, on the other hand, is a very difficult addiction to break, sometimes even in the face of impotence. Some men are able to overcome it, but for others it's necessary to work around the habit and still try to help them restore their sexual function.

IF THERE IS A MEDICAL OR PHYSICAL CAUSE

The first step is, of course, to try to get any illness under control. Men with diabetes, for instance, sometimes come in with a chief complaint of impotence when the real problem is that their diabetes is completely out of control. No one is going to be able to get good erections with a blood-sugar level of 400, for example. Similarly, if a man has hypothyroidism, it's readily treatable. Excess prolactin can often be treated very simply by medication, as well.

But what if your problem is due to a chronic condition, such as arteriosclerosis or long-standing diabetes or hypertension? These are really some of the most common causes of impotence. Not too many years ago, if you had erection difficulties due to a medical illness such as one of these, it was thought that the only treatment available to you was surgery and a penile implant.

Things have changed tremendously since then. There's nothing wrong with a penile implant if you need one. They have been used for a long time, and they do work. Many types of treatments can be tried, however, before implant surgery is considered, beginning with oral medications and moving on to injections of medication into your penis and to mechanical erection-aid devices.

It's now time to discuss all the active treatments that you may be able to use to help you overcome erection difficulties.

ORAL MEDICATIONS (INCLUDING VIAGRA)

As covered earlier, probably the first choice to start with for most men with erection problems is *Viagra*. We discussed Viagra extensively in an earlier chapter, and it would probably be good for you to review that chapter now. Viagra has revolutionized the treatment of impotence. It's easy and simple to use: one pill when needed. It works for up to three-quarters of men with erection problems.

The side effects of Viagra are relatively minor and transient for most people (stuffed-up nose, foggy feeling, headache, stomach upset, flushing, and visual disturbances for a few). However some people, those who take nitroglycerines or other nitrate medications for angina, cannot take Viagra because the combination of Viagra with these angina medications can drop the blood pressure to very dangerous, possibly fatal, levels.

One of the disadvantages of Viagra is that it requires a little planning, as it is necessary to take the medicine thirty minutes to an hour before you plan to make love. If you take it on an empty stomach, the wait will be shorter. If you take it after a large, fatty meal, it could take over an hour to reach effective blood levels.

Another disadvantage is cost. Each pill is fairly expensive, although some patients cut the cost by getting a larger pill and breaking it in half (which is not authorized by the manufacturer).

There are other oral medications that have been noted to help erections and that have been around for many years. They include, especially, (1) *trazodone*, an antidepressant that was discovered by accident to help men with erections when some young men, on high doses, developed erections that wouldn't go down, and (2) *yohimbine*, originally an herbal medicine isolated from the bark of the African yohimbe tree but now a pharmaceutical, produced in reliable strengths by several pharmaceutical companies. This medication does improve erections for some men and is relatively inexpensive. I would definitely recommend, though, that you get it by prescription at a pharmacy rather than obtaining a capsule of unknown strength and purity over the counter. A common trade name is Yocon. It also can be combined with low-dose Viagra (consult your doctor first).

Trazodone seems to work on the central nervous system to help erections, and yohimbine is a peripheral stimulator, working as an alpha blocker and smooth-muscle relaxer. Yohimbine can have a side effect of causing jitteriness and anxiety in some people, especially on first use.

These second-line oral medications may be helpful in perhaps a third of impotent patients. They don't work with the power of Viagra, but they can cause at least partial improvements in sexual functioning when they are successful.

If a man who has soft, poorly maintained erections experiences a 30 percent improvement with one of these medications, this may be enough to make his erections quite adequate for intercourse. Another man who has little or no erection activity to start with might not experience enough improvement from the medications to be noticeable. On the other hand, there might be enough partial improvement for him to be able to have intercourse on occasion with a semierect or three-quarters-erect penis, which still might be an only partially acceptable solution, or he might experience a return of full erections.

There are also some new oral medications *under development* and working their way through the FDA approval process. These include oral *phentolamine*, which only works in perhaps 40 percent of impotent men compared to Viagra's 75 percent but has the advantage of being very inexpensive in comparison with Viagra. Phentolamine also doesn't interact with nitrates. Its primary side effect can be low blood pressure in some cases.

A second impotence drug now under development is *apomorphine*. This medication may turn out to be less promising because of more prominent side effects.

In addition, Pfizer, the makers of Viagra, are working on derivatives of Viagra that may have less interaction with nitrates and/or which may have a faster onset of action.

Another medication treatment involves the use of the male hormone *testosterone*. If your levels of this hormone are deficient, receiving treatment by skin patches or injections may be extremely helpful, especially in conjunction with one or more of the other medications. For more information read over the extensive discussion in chapter 22.

There are herbal remedies that are sometimes recommended for the treatment of impotence, including *ginseng* and *ginkgo biloba*. These medications may be quite valuable for improving one's sense of well-being, but they are not a practical, everyday treatment for impotence in the same way we think of Viagra. They simply don't work that way.

INTRA-URETHRAL MEDICATIONS

The intra-urethral medication currently on the market is *Muse (alprostadil)*. "Intra-urethral" means that you insert this medicine inside the opening of your penis with a little applicator about ten minutes prior to intercourse. It produces an erection in about 40 to 60 percent of men with impotence, which is less than the approximately 75 to 80 percent with Viagra, but it may work for some men for whom Viagra doesn't work, and vice versa. It is obviously less convenient than taking a pill, but on the other hand, its timing is more convenient than Viagra as you don't have to wait thirty to sixty minutes.

The most prominent side effect that patients experience with Muse is pain in the penis, testicles, or groin (which may be intense) in up to a third of patients. Low blood pressure, causing feelings of faintness, or even actual fainting, is another less frequent side effect. Priapism is possible but infrequent.

Muse can cause mild vaginal itching or burning for your partner in about 6 percent of cases.

TOPICAL MEDICATIONS

A form of this same medicine, alprostadil, which could be simply rubbed on the penis, is under development. The advantage is convenience. A medicine that can simply be put on like a cream and produce an erection would obviously be easier to use than one that is inserted into your penis with an applicator. The problem is that it would still have the same potential side effects, pain and hypotension.

One problem with this and other creams and gels under development is that they could conceivably be absorbed from the penis onto your partner's vagina. The possible side effects that the woman partner could experience would have to be studied as well.

PENILE INJECTIONS

Another possibility is penile injecions. This treatment is not as scary as it sounds. It involves the injection of a very small amount of a blood vessel dilator directly into the corpora cavernosa of your penis with a very tiny needle. The corpora cavernosa are the chambers that expand and fill with blood to produce an erection.

In most cases, these injections produce an erection within ten minutes. The erection usually lasts about an hour. You can learn how to administer the injections at home yourself. This treatment is probably successful in 85 to 90 percent of cases.

Currently there are four types of injections in use. The first is *papaverine,* the second is a mixture of *papaverine and phentolamine,* the third is *alprostadil,* and the fourth is a *combination of all three.*

Your doctor can tell you the advantages and disadvantages of the different combinations, but briefly, as you might expect, the combination of all three has the best success rate but also may have more side effects. Alprostadil has gone through the FDA approval system and thus is more expensive than the others. The combination that includes alprostadil is also more expensive. Alprostadil is the same ingredient that causes pain in patients taking Muse, and it also may cause pain when used for penile injections.

The advantages of penile injections compared to Viagra are first that the injections work within ten minutes, second that they are cheaper, and third that they may work for some men for whom Viagra doesn't.

Unfortunately, there are also some drawbacks. The first is the very fact of injections into the penis—an act some men find painful even to contemplate. It's harder still actually to stick a needle, small as it is, into your penis. There can also be some side effects, such as pain, priapism (an erection that won't go down and requires immediate treatment), and possible scarring and Peyronie's disease from multiple injections over many years into the same area of the penis. Priapism, scarring, and Peyronie's are rare but can occur.

Most men who were using the penile injections switched over to Viagra when it came out, but some men have continued to use the injections because of the convenience of having an erection in ten minutes, because of the lower cost, and because the injections work well and the patients are reluctant to change to something new.

MECHANICAL ERECTION AID DEVICES

These devices are basically a plastic cylinder that you place over your penis. You then use a little hand-operated suction pump to create a vacuum and draw blood into your penis. Finally, a heavy rubber band traps the blood in the penis and keeps you erect.

The advantage of this method is that it is probably the safest of all the treatments. The only limitation is that you shouldn't keep it on more than a half hour. (If someone is drunk and passes out with the rubber band on, the lack of circulation could cause gangrene of the penis.)

This is probably also the cheapest of the treatments. Once you've bought the device, successive uses don't cost anything.

Disadvantages include some possible but minor discomfort from the suction and then from the rubber band. The other major disadvantage is aesthetic and practical: This is just not the kind of thing you would slip into your jacket pocket when you go out on a date. This makes these vacuum/constriction devices most suitable for a man in a long-standing, stable relationship with an understanding partner. For someone who is divorced, widowed, or single and dating a number of different women, such an aid may just not be practical.

VASCULAR SURGERY

Vascular surgery for impotence is usually reserved for young men who have suffered some traumatic injury to the penis causing obstruction of the blood supply to the penis, which is preventing erection. The operation bypasses the obstruction in the blood supply, much like a cardiac bypass operation.

Unfortunately, though, the blood vessels are smaller, the surgery more difficult, and the results less successful with older men than with cardiac bypasses. That is why this surgery is usually reserved for younger men who may have suffered some traumatic injury impairing their blood supply, but who are presumed to have less arteriosclerosis in their small blood vessels. On the right candidate and with a surgeon who has had lots of experience with this kind of operation the results may be successful in 75 percent of cases.

Expensive penile arteriograms and other studies of your penile circulation are not warranted as part of an impotence evaluation unless vascular surgery is seriously contemplated.

PENILE IMPLANTS

As you can see, there are many possible treatments for impotence. Some men don't respond to any of them, however, usually because their vascular supply or corpora cavernosa are too damaged by a disease such as diabetes or by treatment for prostate cancer.

If the treatments we've discussed above don't work for you, a surgical implant probably will be recommended. Penile implant operations are quite common, safe, and successful. And they work! They are an excellent alternative for a man who wants to maintain his erection ability but has not responded to the other means of treatment outlined here. I'll tell you more about implants in the next chapter.

TREATMENT FOR
PREMATURE EJACULATION

Premature ejaculation, or coming too quickly, is a problem that mostly affects younger men. Older men usually require longer stimulation before thay can climax. Occasionally, however, this problem does affect older men. If you suffer from this problem, it can be very frustrating, both for you and for your partner.

A class of medications, the SSRIs, which are a type of antidepressants, were discovered to have a side effect of delaying ejaculation. Although this can be a problem for some people, for a man with premature ejaculation it can be a blessing. If you have this problem, a trial with at least one of these medications, which include Prozac, Zoloft, Paxil, and others, would be worthwhile.

Other older men come too quickly due to unconsciously hurrying because they are afraid of losing their erection. In other words, they are thinking to themselves, "Oh, my God! It's going to go down!" and they come without wanting to. For men with this problem, a trial with Viagra will give them the assurance that their erection will stay and thus they may be able to keep from coming.

CHAPTER 26

THE PENILE IMPLANT

What It Is and How It Works

I n the last chapter I discussed the wide range of nonsurgical treatments currently available for men with impotence. Unfortunately, as I pointed out at the end of the chapter, they don't work for everyone. However, there is a treatment, well tested and widely used, that can enable you to have erections again, at any age, no matter what the cause of your impotence. This is the penile implant.

You should not consider getting a penile implant as your initial treatment. As this is a surgical treatment, you should try at least one, and probably several, of the treatments discussed in the previous chapter before giving up and getting an implant.

Patients tend to have many questions about penile implants. Some men arrive at the doctor's office knowing exactly what a penile implant is, and they've already decided that it's what they want. Other men, on the contrary, are certain they don't want surgery under any circumstances. Some men, not really sure what a penile implant actually is, tend to think in terms of what they've read about heart transplants, for instance, or artificial limbs.

A penile implant is *not* an artificial penis that replaces your own. It's not a transplant like a heart transplant or a corneal transplant. A penile implant is simply a replacement of the erection mechanism of your own penis.

The implant, consisting of two silicone-covered cylinders, is surgically inserted into your penis in much the way a breast implant is placed within a woman's breast in an enlargement operation. Just as the breast implant leaves the external appearance of the breast unchanged except for the increase in size, a penile implant inside your penis doesn't appreciably alter its outward appearance. If you could have climaxes and ejaculate before you had the implant, you should be able to do so afterward. You can even father a child.

HOW YOUR ERECTION MECHANISM NORMALLY WORKS

Under normal circumstances, you get an erection when blood fills two long, spongy cylinders, the corpora cavernosa, that run the length of your penis. Your erection becomes firm and hard in much the same way that a long, cylindrical balloon becomes stiff when you inflate it. Later, when the blood drains from your penis, the erection deflates.

This erection mechanism can be very fragile, as it requires your vascular and nervous systems to work together in a complicated fashion. Many different factors can cause it to work irregularly or not at all. If your erection system isn't working and it can't be restored by medication or other nonsurgical means, it can be replaced by penile implants inserted into your corpora cavernosa.

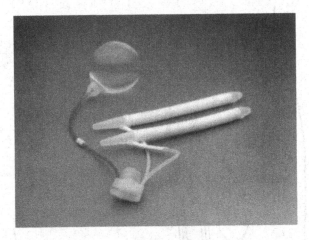

Figure 26-1. Three-part inflatable implant. Courtesy of American Medical Systems, Inc.

THE DIFFERENT KINDS OF IMPLANTS

There are four basic types, the first of which is called *the three-part inflatable implant* (see Figures 26-1 and 26-2). This device very accurately mimics your normal erection process. Two empty silicone-covered cylindrical balloons are implanted in the corpora cavernosa of your penis. When you want to have an erection, you squeeze a tiny pump implanted in your scrotum. This forces a saline fluid from a reservoir behind your pubic bone into the expandable balloons in your penis. The fluid causes your penis to extend and expand into a nearly normal erection (see Figures 26-3 and 26-4).

After using the erection, you can press a little release valve on the pump. The balloons will deflate, the fluid returns to the reservoir, and your penis returns to its limp state. Accidental deflation won't occur unless there's a mechanical breakdown of some kind.

The second type of implant is called the *two-part inflatable implant.* It consists of the same inflatable cylinders, but the pump

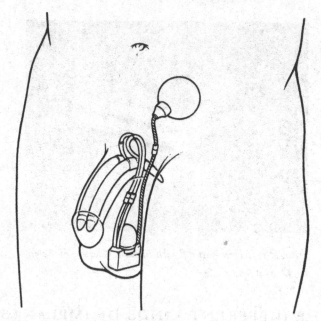

Figure 26-2. Three-part inflatable implant. Courtesy of American Medical Systems, Inc.

and resevoir are combined in a single unit and inserted in your scrotum (see Figures 26-5 and 26-6).

The next type is the *self-contained inflatable implant*. In this model the pump and the reservoir are all contained as a single unit in the cylinders. This allows them to be implanted entirely within the penis. Its appearance is similar to the flexible implant, which we describe in the next paragraph.

The *flexible implant* is the simplest of all those that are currently in fairly widespread use. It's not inflatable at all but consists of flexible, silicon-covered cylinders surrounding an inner core made of braided silver or stainless-steel wire. You can straighten it into an erect position for intercourse or bend it down, out of the way, when an erection is not needed. The bendable braided wire core lets it stay in the position that you put it in (see Figure 26-7).

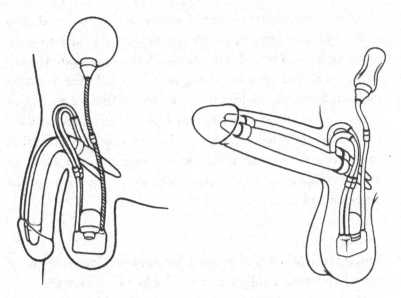

Figures 26-3 and 26-4. Three-part inflatable implant. Courtesy of American Medical Systems, Inc.

Now that we are familiar with the principles according to which these devices work, let's examine the advantages and disadvantages of each.

The Three-Part Inflatable Implant   The inflatable implant consists of two expandable silicone balloons surgically inserted into the erectile tubes of your penis. You don't feel them once the surgery heals any more than a woman feels the implants in her breasts.

The implants are connected to a small reservoir balloon inserted in the fatty tissue of your abdomen just in front of your bladder. A tiny pump hangs in your scrotum, above your testicles. The implant is cosmetically unnoticeable. There is no scar on your penis, because the incision is on your abdomen or scrotum. The penis looks normal in both the erect and flaccid states.

There is a potential problem, however, in that you are dealing with a rather complex hydraulic system that is subject to occasional mechanical breakdowns. Although these breakdowns aren't serious (a kinked piece of tubing or a fluid leak, for instance), they usually require reoperation to be fixed. About 2 percent of patients will undergo reoperation each year to repair one of these minor mechanical failures. This can be annoying, uncomfortable, and expensive, and there can be some danger, however slight, of surgical complications. Let's review both the pros and cons of the three-part inflatable.

Advantages

This is the gold standard of inflatable implants. It gives the most natural-appearing result. Your penis looks like a naturally functioning penis, and your erections resemble normal erections.

Besides just being erect, your penis actually fills out in width and becomes full. This doesn't happen with the flexible implants, and it happens only slightly with the self-contained inflatable rods. With the two-part inflatables there is more expansion than the self-contained, but less than the three-part because, with the combined pump/reservoir in your scrotum, there is simply less fluid in the reservoir.

There's no problem with concealment. The scar is not visible. The erection is flaccid when you're not using it. The implant is relatively undetectable—and comfortable.

Disadvantages

It requires more difficult, longer surgery and more skill and experience on the part of the surgeon. Get these done by a surgeon who does lots of them and is very familiar with the surgery, not one who does them just once in a while.

Mechanical failures may necessitate reoperation.

The costs of both the implant and the surgery are greater than for the one- and two-part implants.

The Two-Part Inflatable Implant This implant consists of the inflatable silicon-covered balloons in the penis but the reservoir, instead of being a separate balloon in the lower abdomen, is combined with the pump in the scrotum. Again, there is no scar on your penis. The hydraulic system is simpler, with fewer, and shorter, tubes carrying fluid here and there than the three-part.

Advantages

It's easier to put in than the three-part. It requires less skill by the surgeon. It's less expensive.

Disadvantages

What goes in the scrotum, the combination pump and reservoir, is necessarily considerably larger than the simple pump that you

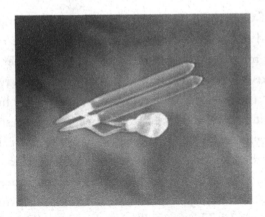

Figure 26-5. Two-part inflatable implant. Courtesy of Mentor Corp.

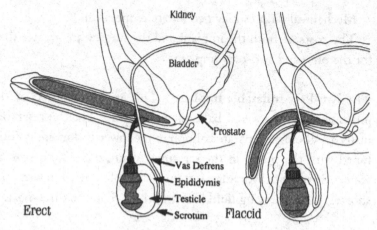

Figure 26-6. Two-part inflatable implant. Courtesy of Mentor Corp.

have with the three-part implant. Therefore, it's more obvious and easier to detect.

Erection is less satisfactory because of less expansion of width and fullness. Flaccidity is less complete and less natural-looking.

The Self-Contained Inflatable Implant   This implant has a pump and reservoir mechanism included within the rod itself. It works by moving fluid from one part of the cylinder to another part where it is held more tightly and thus produces rigidity.

When the implant is not inflated, your penis hangs down limply, but because the fluid and the mechanism are still both inside the cylinders, your penis doesn't have the total limpness of the empty balloon of the three-part inflatable implant.

When you want to use the inflatable rod, you squeeze a pump on the rod, within or just behind the head of your penis, depending on the model. This forces fluid within the cylinder into a non-expandable inner cylinder that inflates and becomes firm. Just part

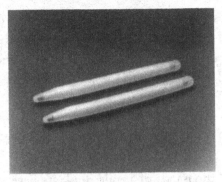

Figure 26-7. The Flexible/Malleable Implant. Courtesy of American Medical Systems, Inc.

of the inflatable rod, therefore, actually inflates. You deflate it by pressing a valve on the cylinder itself.

Advantages
Compared to the three-part implant, it involves much easier surgery and is much cheaper. There are also fewer possibilities for mechanical breakdowns.

Disadvantages
There is, of course, a less natural limpness, less expansion of girth with erection, and a less satisfactory erection overall.

The Flexible/Malleable Implant   This silicon-covered cylinder can be bent into shape, and it will stay in that shape because of its inner core of braided silver wire. This implant has a lot of the same advantages and disadvantages as the self-contained inflatable. It has the same surgical simplicity, decreased expense, and relative lack of mechanical problems. There is no expansion or filling out at all with erection, though. And, after a long period of time, it is possible for the silver wires in the flexible implant to wear out and break from constantly being bent back and forth. The implant then would lose its ability to keep the position it is bent into and would return to the constantly erect position.

WHO USES PENILE IMPLANTS?

Hundreds of thousands of penile implants have been used successfully. They are clearly far from experimental.

Approximately three-quarters of the men who have received penile implants are between the ages of forty and seventy. However, men as young as nineteen or twenty have received implants because of erection inability due to accidents or medical illness, and men in their eighties have also received them. About 10 percent of implants are given to men older than seventy years of age.

Men most commonly require penile implants because of impotence from diabetes, vascular disease, certain types of prostate or rectal surgery, pelvic nerve injury, and spinal cord injury.

As we wrote earlier in the chapter, a penile implant probably shouldn't be considered until you have tried nonsurgical treatments such as Viagra and found them ineffective.

WHAT KIND OF OPERATION IS REQUIRED?

As mentioned before, the most complicated and lengthy surgery is required for the three-part inflatable implant. It will take about an hour and a half to two hours, as opposed to about forty-five minutes to an hour for one of the self-contained implants. The incidence of postoperative infection is only about 1.5 percent for all types of implants.

The average hospital stay for a patient recuperating from an inflatable implant is usually just one day. For a one-piece implant, some of the procedures are actually performed on an outpatient surgery basis.

The overall success rate with all kinds of implants is in the range of 95 percent, but this varies depending on the skill and expertise of the individual surgeon involved.

You will probably be told to wait for three to six weeks before having intercourse. Most patients do wait close to six weeks. A small number of patients (probably fewer than 5 percent) have some degree of pain continuing for a time after surgery. In almost all cases, this eventually disappears.

HOW SATISFIED ARE MEN AND THEIR PARTNERS WITH THE RESULTS?

Reaction seems to be very positive. Most men report good sensation and enjoyable lovemaking with an implant, particularly with the inflatable varieties.

About 75 to 90 percent of men who receive penile implants seem to be satisfied with their sexual responses. Most female partners of men who have received implants report that they would recommend the operation to a couple considering it if the man needs it.

If a man's partner is positive about lovemaking, her response to an implant will probably be very good. Rather than feeling uncomfortable with the idea, most women tend to be quite happy with their partners' new potency. But it's important to have realistic expectations: If your female partner is negative about sex before you have an implant, your having an implant probably won't change her attitude.

Men who were impotent but now have an implant generally experience an improvement in self-esteem, knowing that they can now have sexual relations. Even single men who do little dating and only use their implants infrequently say that just knowing that they are capable of having intercourse is very important to them. They feel more comfortable with women, knowing that if a situation led to a romantic sexual encounter, they would have the capacity to perform.

IN SUMMARY

A penile implant can make an enormous difference to a man who has erection problems but doesn't respond to other forms of treatment. If you are one of these men, you have the opportunity to continue an active sex life indefinitely. Aside from your own enjoyment, this can give you the self-esteem of continuing to please your partner, as well as the warmth and intimacy that a continued loving and sexual relationship can bring.

CONCLUSION

CHAPTER 27

RECAPTURING INTENSITY

Keeping a long-term relationship fresh is a problem all couples face. We seek out long-term relationships for the security and comfort they provide, yet we want our sexual relations to feel new, fresh, and exciting. The question is how we can maintain newness, freshness, and continuing intensity in a sexual relationship that is no longer new.

This dilemma does not have one single solution. Some couples abandon the attempt and either let sex die out completely or continue a lovemaking pattern marked by day-to-day sameness and repetition. This may mean making love once a week, in the same place, on the same day, and in the same way. It's all over in ten minutes, from start to finish. It isn't awful or unpleasant, just uninteresting and unexciting.

Some partners who are unhappy either with the demise of their sexual lives or with continuing sexual monotony look for sexual contacts outside of marriage. Some cultures have made mistresses or extramarital lovers practically an accepted solution to the problem of sexual boredom.

It doesn't have to be this way. Continued lovemaking in a long-term relationship can be more satisfying and more interesting than that in any brief relationship. Sex therapist Dr. Ruth Westheimer states this beautifully in *Dr. Ruth's Guide to Good Sex:*

> There may be too much talk about sex in marriages or long relationships getting dull. I want to explain that it isn't the nature of the thing to be boring. Long sexual relationships offer pleasures you can't get any other way. Making love with the partner you have had for twenty years, who knows you better than anyone else, who has shared life's ups and downs with you, can be a royal pleasure.

If your sexual relationship has become dull, reestablishing intensity and excitement won't come automatically. It will require time and effort on your part. It's most likely to succeed if you and your partner have feelings of true affection for each other and a genuine interest in improving your sexual lives.

It's crucial to see yourselves as "lovers" again as well as "husband" and "wife." If your relationship has settled into dull marriage roles and you've stopped feeling like lovers, you may start to see both your partner and yourself as drab and unsexual. When you treat each other as household fixtures, sex can become blah. This can make an outside sex interest, which gives you or your partner the feeling of being exciting again, very inviting.

The concept of not seeing yourself *just* as husband and wife is very important. In our society, the role of "husband" or "wife" has an entirely different emotional tone than that of "lover." The terms *husband* and *wife* imply reliability, solidity, security, duties, and responsibilities. *Lover* implies excitement, allure, passion, romance, play, fun, and, of course, love.

Now don't misunderstand me. You want, *you need to have*, those solid husband and wife qualities in a long-term relationship. But if you have *only* these qualities, your relationship may be solid but it may also be dull. In addition to security and responsibility, you need to regain the romance and excitement of being lovers again as well.

I'd like to suggest that you talk with your partner about how the two of you can get back that feeling of being lovers. Make it clear that he or she is special to you and valued and cherished. And don't make it clear only with words. Show your affection with caresses, hugs, and kisses, especially at times when it's not a prelude to lovemaking. Also tell your partner about the qualities you most appreciate in him or her. It's so easy, in a long-term relationship, to assume, "Oh, he [or she] already knows I appreciate that."

Get back that feeling of discovery and excitement in your relationship. Plan unusual vacations or projects; continuing to have adventures together is a way of keeping your lives interesting.

Reestablish some of those activities you remember from your courting days. Go out dancing, go to a restaurant, or to movies or the theater together. Remember the flowers and little gifts that can give extra expressions of love. Don't save romance for special occasions like anniversaries or birthdays.

One important but infrequently thought of step is putting a muzzle on your television set. Keeping it on all evening, every evening, can do more to make your lives dull and dampen your love life than almost anything else. Watching late-night TV especially can be terribly destructive to possible lovemaking opportunities, as you are likely to turn it off only when you are really fatigued and thoughts of sex have gone by the wayside.

If there's a program coming on late in the evening that you feel you must watch, consider making love in the early evening, before it comes on. Then you can watch your program with a nice sexual glow. Or else, record the program on a VCR so you can watch it at your leisure.

Up to this point I have talked about what you can do to get back some of the *feelings* in your relationship. Making your *lovemaking* interesting and exciting again is another question.

DISCUSS THIS CHAPTER WITH YOUR PARTNER

You and your partner should really review this chapter together; it will take commitment from each of you to recapture the feeling of being lovers again.

Making love at the same old time and in predictable ways may be monotonous, but it also brings a certain sense of security. This sense of security that comes from familiar routine causes inertia and resistance to change. Breaking out of this rut will be exciting and gratifying, but it will take effort and initiative from both of you.

MAKE YOUR LOVEMAKING A HIGH PRIORITY

You must decide that being a lover to your partner is important in your life—more important, in fact, than most of your day-to-day activities. Lovemaking has to rank above doing the dishes, balancing the checkbook, or doing some extra paperwork you brought home from the office. Don't put off making love in order to start last-minute chores that don't have to be done right away. It's not something to save until you're tired at the end of a long day, when your body is telling you that it's time to go to sleep.

HUG AND CARESS IN BED EVEN IF YOU'RE NOT PLANNING TO MAKE LOVE

Don't feel that bedtime caressing is only for the nights when you ~~ planning to make love. Set aside some time before going to ~~~ it's just a minute or two, for affection. It doesn't have to ~~~~~~~ ~~ddle every night, you won't necessarily make love mor~~ ~~~~~'ll certainly both feel more loved and loving.

VARY WHEN AND WHERE YOU MAKE LOVE

Try making love at different times of the day. Go back to bed after breakfast, if you have the opportunity, or have a romantic lovemaking session in the middle of the afternoon with the sun streaming in your window.

Try making love in different places in your house as well. Consider the living-room couch, or throw a quilt over some soft carpeting or a throw rug on the floor.

Plan an occasional night for a special romantic atmosphere. Use candles and music, perhaps a special wine, a fire in the fireplace—whatever your imagination comes up with. Planning together is fun, but don't overlook the delight that surprise can bring.

Let yourself be open to spontaneous lovemaking. If your partner suggests lovemaking at an unusual time, or when you aren't expecting it, or when you have other plans or other things on your mind, don't say no automatically. Break that negative habit. Let yourself feel young again—make love right on the spot. You may find it truly exhilarating.

VARY LOVEMAKING TECHNIQUES AND POSITIONS

Discuss new petting and caressing techniques with your partner. Think how you can vary standard ways of caressing by starting on a different part of your partner's body, such as fingertips or toes. Try caressing each other with sensuous fabrics such as silk or satin, or use a feather brush, or try caressing with body oils.

Be adventurous. Try new lovemaking positions. If you usually make love with the woman lying on her back, try some variations. Let her bring her knees all the way up, wrap her legs around the man's waist, or bring them up over his shoulders. (She will feel a different kind of vaginal stimulation with her pelvis tilted like this.)

Try making love with the woman kneeling on top, or lying on her stomach with a pillow under her pelvis, or kneeling at the edge of the bed while her partner enters her from behind. Let your imaginations run freely. Invent some positions of your own.

GIVE YOUR PARTNER ALL THE WONDERFUL FEELINGS YOU CAN IMAGINE

Before lovemaking, try to imagine how you would like your partner to feel at the height of sexual excitement. Then concentrate on how you can give your partner all those delightful and wonderful feelings.

Think, too, of lovemaking as play. Give yourselves permission to be silly, curious, foolish, and joyful. Lovemaking isn't work, and it doesn't have to be serious.

YOU WILL BOTH FEEL EXCITED ABOUT THE VARIETY IN YOUR LOVEMAKING

I realize that you can't keep discovering totally new ways of love-making every time, but that's not really the goal I'm suggesting. Rather, I'm trying to help you find ways to overcome a serious danger in all long-term sexual relationships: the danger of mo-notony.

If you use a variety of different caresses, different ⌐s, different music, occasional lubricants or oils, and different ⌐ for sex, you will, of course, repeat yourself in time, but your lov⌐ life certainly won't be boring. You'll be able to capture that sense of novelty and excitement that adds such spice to sex. If the two of you work together, discuss this chapter, and plan a new rela-tionship together, you *can* change your lives.

TRYING NEW PATTERNS OF LOVEMAKING

A remarkable number of the older couples I see in my practice seem to be stuck on the idea that there's only one appropriate pat-tern for lovemaking—the one they've been following. Often this consists of a certain amount of foreplay leading to intercourse, during which the man climaxes.

While some couples realistically expect that the woman will

usually climax with clitoral stimulation, either before or after intercourse, a surprising number in this day and age still feel that the only valid way for the woman to climax is during intercourse. For them, lovemaking ends when the man climaxes or loses his erection. If she hasn't climaxed by then, they rarely make an attempt to have her do so by manual or oral stimulation.

Often it's the woman herself who feels that climaxing outside of intercourse isn't natural or makes her uncomfortable. She'll say she only wants to climax the "natural" way, and thus she refuses or is reluctant to have her partner help her climax manually or orally.

What these couples consider "unnatural"—climaxing from manual or oral clitoral stimulation—is actually the natural way of climaxing for the majority of women. Female sexual response certainly seems to be designed for this method of stimulation. For an older couple to insist on mandatory climaxes during intercourse for both the man and the woman puts tremendous pressure on a man with a possibly already fragile erection reflex. If he doesn't get fully erect or doesn't maintain his erection, his partner remains frustrated—and he feels like a failure.

One particular couple in their middle fifties related the wide variety of lovemaking patterns they had used on a single weekend. They had used these patterns not to be eccentric or outrageous, but simply to be comfortable and to adapt in a natural way to some of the changes of aging. I'll let Betty tell you about their experience:

> Bill and I were thinking about the different ways we made love last weekend. We hadn't planned any particular kind of sex at all. It was just the way it turned out.
>
> So many people we know feel that sex is a failure if it doesn't work out exactly the way it's supposed to—like if both of them don't climax. Bill and I feel that as we've gotten older

we've outgrown that kind of foolishness. We've learned to enjoy our lovemaking for what it is—each time.

For instance, this last Friday we came home late and
tired. We got into bed with neither of us having any idea of
making love. We started playing around a little, though, and we
gradually got turned on. I caressed Bill's penis until he got
hard, and we had intercourse for a little while, and then we
tired out and quit. Neither of us climaxed, but we dropped off
to sleep feeling happy and content.

Saturday morning we could sleep late. We woke up cuddling and Bill started playing with me—first with his hand and
then with his tongue. I just lay back in bed half asleep and enjoyed him licking me. It felt divine.

My arthritis bothers me, though, first thing in the morning. I usually feel stiff when I first wake up, and I can't climax.
So I asked Bill to come up in the bed where I could reach him,
and I used my hand and mouth to get him hard. Then I rolled
over onto my side and he slipped into my vagina from behind.
That's the easiest way for me to get started when my arthritis is
bothering me.

We made love leisurely that way for a while. Then I rolled
over onto my stomach and put a pillow under my hips, and we
just kept on with him on top of me. Finally, when my joints
felt a little looser, I turned over on my back for some more.
Eventually, Bill pulled out. He hadn't come, so I helped him to
finish with my hand. It was fun, watching him come.

You know, we could've spoiled that delightful experience
by finding fault with ourselves—because I hadn't climaxed, and
because Bill didn't climax inside me. We didn't, though. We felt
that our lovemaking was wonderful. We felt warm, close, and
loving all day because of it.

Saturday night while we were in bed talking, Bill started
playing with me again. I hadn't come either that morning or the

night before, so this time I really was ready. He started licking my clitoris with his tongue while his fingers were in my vagina rubbing what I guess is my G-spot. That certainly feels terrific to me, and I climax most easily that way. I had a big climax, which pleased Bill greatly (me, too!).

After resting a minute or two, I started to stroke him. He got partly hard, but he just didn't feel that he needed to come again or have more sex after having come that morning. He suggested we wait until the next day. He felt proud of the nice orgasm he had given me, and we both felt good.

Sunday morning we slept in again. We felt very snuggly and warm and petted each other until I got wet and he got hard, and this time he came inside me.

He offered to pet me to climax too, but I asked him to wait until after breakfast. (My arthritis is always better after I've moved around a bit.) He was glad to wait. We did go back to bed after eggs and bacon, and he had fun bringing me to another wonderful climax. We don't always have so much lovemaking in a weekend, but this one was wonderful.

It wasn't that this couple had "so much" lovemaking, but that they had so many little fragments of lovemaking. They didn't have strict rules, so they accepted whatever aspect of lovemaking happened to come along, and they felt comfortable with it. In fact, none of their lovemaking episodes fit the rigid mythical model of sex: simple intercourse with the man always hard and ready to ejaculate and the woman climaxing during intercourse. But what was really important was that this older couple had truly learned how to appreciate sex and themselves. They were happy each time with whatever happened in their lovemaking, and they weren't critical of their own performance or their partner's. They have really learned what "making love" is all about.

INDEX

ABOUT THE AUTHOR

Saul H. Rosenthal, M.D., is a graduate of Harvard College and Harvard Medical School. Following additional postgraduate training at Harvard, he taught for a number of years at the University of Texas Medical School, where he was an associate professor. Dr. Rosenthal then went into private practice, where he founded the Sexual Therapy Clinic of San Antonio. He also was the founding editor of the *Sex Over 40* newsletter. He is now enjoying retirement with his wife and daughter.